BRENDA KINSEL'S

FASHION MAKEOVER

BRENDA KINSEL'S

FASHION
MAKEOVER

30 DAYS TO DIVA STYLE!

CHRONICLE BOOKS
SAN FRANCISCO

Library of Congress Cataloging-in-Publication Data available.

ISBN - 13: 978 - 0 - 8118 - 5738 - 3
ISBN - 10 : 0 - 8118 - 5738 - 7

Manufactured in China.

Designed by Efrat Rafaeli.
Typesetting by Efrat Rafaeli and Leslie Hendin.

Distributed in Canada by Raincoast Books
9050 Shaughnessy Street
Vancouver, British Columbia V6P 6E5

10 9 8 7 6 5 4 3 2 1

Chronicle Books LLC
680 Second Street
San Francisco, California 94107
www.chroniclebooks.com

To my beautiful Bellas, Lynn Sydney and Marjory DeRoeck

Introduction • **EVERYDAY DIVA**

PAGE 8

Chapter 1 • **IT'S ABOUT TIME**

PAGE 15

Chapter 2 • **WELCOME TO BRENDA'S 30-DAY BEAUTY CAMP**

PAGE 23

WEEK ONE

Chapter 3 • **RUTS**

PAGE 30

Chapter 4 • **RESONANCE**

PAGE 45

Chapter 5 • **COLOR YOUR WORLD**

PAGE 49

Chapter 6 • **DEFINING YOUR DIVA STYLE**

PAGE 61

Chapter 7 • **FIT FOR A DIVA**

PAGE 78

WEEK TWO

Chapter 8 • **TAMING THE CLOSET**

PAGE 98

Chapter 9 • **ACCESSORY NECESSITIES**

PAGE 108

Chapter 10 • **PUTTING IT TOGETHER**

PAGE 122

WEEK THREE

Chapter 11 • **SHOPPING**

PAGE 148

WEEK FOUR

Chapter 12 • **HAIR**

PAGE 166

Chapter 13 • **MAKEUP**

PAGE 176

Chapter 14 • **DIVA DATES**

PAGE 189

Chapter 15 • **DIVA FOREVER**

PAGE 203

Index

PAGE 213

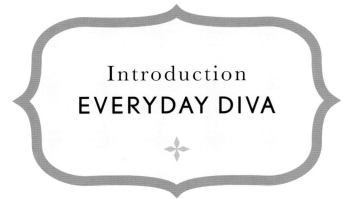

Introduction
EVERYDAY DIVA

I'll never forget the day Stephanie, a client of mine, called with news that gave me a sharp pain in my chest. "Brenda," she said, "my mother was visiting me and she said I should give up on clothes, that clothes are for the young and I should leave fashion to them. It's time to throw in the towel."

"Hold on," I replied. "You sound like you're losing consciousness. I'll be right over!"

I rushed to her house, cornered her in her closet, and said, "Now what's this business about giving up on fashion? Why would you do that?"

"Well, I don't *really* want to give up. But I am over fifty . . ." she said, looking down at the floor.

I made her look at me. "But you've never been more gorgeous!" I exclaimed. I rattled off a list of her assets—her flashing brown eyes and healthy hair, the curves in her waist and hips that screamed sensuality. "It's not over! You're at the height of your brilliance!" I said.

Her eyes flashed. She stood up, her shoulders dropped back, and some fire returned to her voice. She seemed to be pondering her options and then blurted out, "I may be over fifty, but I'm not dead!"

That's right. And if you're reading this right now, you're not dead either. Like Stephanie and every other woman I know who is over thirty-five, you're probably sitting on a heap of accomplishments and accolades—from the revenues you brought to your department at work to the volunteer group you headed that raised money for Hurricane Katrina victims to the kids you've raised who have even thanked you for a job well done. Come on, you're awesome! You're the best you've ever been! Why shouldn't it show in the way you look?

Now, I'm not clueless. I understand that fashion is a difficult path to navigate. It's hard to know what's appropriate if we look in magazines for inspiration. The models weigh as much as a loaf of wheat bread and have faces that are as fresh as the faces of the girls on the junior varsity basketball team. These are not women we can relate to. Against our will, our bodies have decided to redistribute our weight, and suddenly we have breadth where we never had it before. Caught up in the flurry of life, we may have let one, two, or even fifteen years go by when we hardly had a minute to tend to our wardrobes. So when we do walk into a store, it's like entering a nightclub with loud music and a blinding overhead disco ball twirling around and around, making us feel dizzy, overwhelmed, and wanting to find the nearest exit.

Or maybe you've settled on being great on the inside, but you've given up looking fabulous on the outside. Well, let me tell you where I stand on this: As a woman over forty you deserve to revel in your accomplishments and present yourself to the world as a beautiful, confident being.

Let's look at the alternative. If you've been in a fashion slumber for years and have let yourself go, chances are you're looking older than your years. In a word, dowdy. I don't say this to be mean; months or years of neglect add up, and there's a discernible consequence. Does anyone ever want to look dowdy? I don't think so! "Dowdy" means lacking stylishness; it implies a woman is old-fashioned and unattractive. It's not a look someone goes for; it's a look someone defaults to.

There may be many reasons why a vibrant, successful woman defaults to dowdy, including you. It could be you've lost touch with yourself after putting everyone else first for so long. You've forgotten how to spend time on yourself. As a result, the clothes you throw on every day have no spark left in them, your hair hasn't been styled or updated in months, and your makeup routine is uninspired. Or maybe you just never figured out how to put a look together from head to toe and diverted your attention to something you could conquer. Or maybe you never valued style to begin with. Instead, you focused on your intellectual and spiritual development, and your contributions to social causes. Here's a news flash: There are women who value all those things and have beauty and style, too. You can be one of them, and I'm here to show you how.

Whether you see it in the mirror or not, there's a lot that has gone into shaping who you are. Let's use it all! By looking at your passions, personality, and lifestyle, we'll come up with the formula to express your true self. Don't worry. I'm not going to try to wedge you into a micromini or convince you that you can wear only taupe. Instead, I'm going to help you determine what looks best on you.

If you don't identify yourself as a woman with diva style, think again. You've followed your heart along with your head. You've been over rough spots and come out the other end. You're better than ever. That's why I'm using the word *diva* to describe you. It is big enough to contain all of you—your personality, your values, your passions.

Let me explain. *Diva* is the Italian word for "goddess," a woman of great beauty or grace. We often think of a diva as a woman with a fabulous singing voice and a captivating and commanding stage presence. Here's how I see it: A diva is a woman at the top of her game. She's ripe and juicy, free to love, and open to receiving it. She's aware of her talents and gifts, and she uses them. She's not afraid to shine and distinguish herself from others. A diva is the star of her life but doesn't diminish others. In fact, she inspires greatness. She doesn't play games, is honest and up-front. We trust her. A handful of divas come immediately to mind—Goldie Hawn, Diane Sawyer, Oprah, Queen Latifah.

Sure, *diva* can also have a negative connotation, but I'm not talking about a temperamental diva or someone with a demanding "look at me" persona. The diva I'm thinking

of is someone who expresses herself confidently through her beauty and style. That someone can be you.

While you're on the road from dowdy to diva, I'm going to encourage you to express yourself clearly, climb out of your fashion and dressing ruts, and create habits of self care. I'll teach you how to articulate your current style so you can put a look together from head to toe. I plan to help you get rid of the things in your closet and your makeup drawer that are making you look dated and old. And then, with the help of other Diva Advisors I've brought with me, I'm going to teach you how to care for yourself so you can look sharp and put together whenever you want to.

And you're going to do it in thirty days. That's right, this program aims to shape up your wardrobe in a few short weeks. To make it interesting and to keep you focused on the prize—looking like the diva you really are—you'll plan to go on three dates dressed in your new diva style when the program ends. There will be help all along the way as you dump the dowdy duds from two decades ago, shop for the elements of your three great outfits, and put them together. I even have a Diva Advisor to help you plan the dates! You'll be fabulous, mind-blowingly fabulous. I promise.

Let's get back to Stephanie, who had considered giving up on dressing stylishly. We had a heart-to-heart about the things she loved about her wardrobe. Then we talked about what wasn't working—trying to fit into pants when her body just wasn't suited to them, and wearing stiff fabrics when her curves loved flowing fabrics. I encouraged Stephanie to accept the silhouettes that worked best for her and let go of the mistakes in her closet. We agreed that she was a vibrant woman and deserved to dress that way, in sensual fabrics, beautiful prints, and luxurious wraps. We moved the dowdy items out of her wardrobe—the things that didn't fit any longer, were of inferior quality, or failed in some way to meet her diva standards. They needed to go so she could see the diva pieces that were already in her closet. I wrapped her in fabrics and color combinations that spoke to her ultrafeminine, sexy self—flirty floral silk chiffon skirts, luxurious apricot silk tops, and textured jackets. To complete her look, she wore bold jewelry that added luster and sheen and brought light to her face. Dowdy? No way! Diva? Yes, in Stephanie's way.

Maybe with all this talk about divas, you've been noticing a compressed, tight feeling in your belly. This is your potential to shine, which you may have been stifling for years. It's ready to burst out, and you're unable or unwilling to hold it back any longer. Hooray! Now, at last, no matter what condition your figure is in or how much money is in your bank account, you are finally ready to take the spotlight in your life.

Every woman can be a diva. You don't have to be a size 2 or have straight hair. You don't have to be six feet tall. Divas come in all shapes and sizes, and they aren't limited to the entertainment business. They are what I like to call "everyday divas." If you look, you may find them at the meetings you attend, the class you're enrolled in, or at the office.

• Flowing fabrics make Stephanie an everyday diva.

Does Stephanie's story inspire you as it does me? Do you want to introduce a greater sense of style to your appearance? If you're feeling out of touch with yourself and how you look, feel blah or invisible, or just don't know how to put it all together, this book will show you the way.

The plan is simple to follow, and best of all, it's fun. Before you begin, you'll take a day to clear any obstacles—both the mental ones and the ones on your calendar. Then, in Week One, you're going to learn how to wear colors that look good on you and make you feel good. You'll discover your current diva style and learn how clothes should fit you now. In Week Two you'll be editing your closet and putting great outfits together. Week Three will be devoted to shopping. During Week Four, you'll be off to get hair and makeup ready for your three dates. Afterward, you'll have a chance to reflect on how far you've come and where you'd like to go from here as you continue to explore your unique self.

If this 30-day plan takes you 60 or 90 days, that's okay, too. Every step you take will make a significant difference in how you look and feel and how others see you. Whether you're going out shopping, meeting a girlfriend, or attending a play, you will look as if you've truly arrived.

You'll meet several Diva Advisors along the way who will help you with special issues. The first one, Carole Ann Lyons, is a marketing guru who knows the importance of being up-to-date. In a sense, you're going to be reinventing yourself at this juicy time of your life, and she's here to set you up with tips on how to do that.

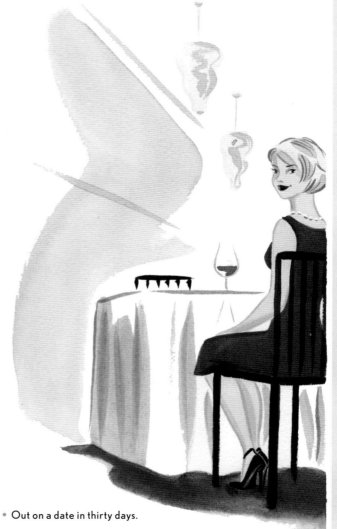

• Out on a date in thirty days.

HOW TO REINVENT YOURSELF

BY Carole Ann Lyons

✦

Carole Ann Lyons has reinvented herself through a variety of top-level careers in publishing, retail marketing, and direct marketing. She is currently called the creative maniac at MillerMania, a video production and marketing company that she cofounded in Camino, California, in 1996. It is, she says, her best reinvention.

Aspiring divas everywhere, fess up: The very idea of having to reinvent ourselves sends us off to bed with the covers pulled tightly up over our heads. The thought of change is so unsettling. Who wants to be jolted out of her comfort zone?

Some of us are even caught up in a complicated style time warp. We are locked into a period when our lives were ticking along like perfect clocks with everything in sync: hair, makeup, body image, wardrobe, friends, lovers, the works. We think, "Wow, this has always worked. Why change a thing?" Instead of continuing to develop our personal image, we stop dead in our tracks, assuming it's too risky to evolve and change. It's as if we suddenly stopped in time.

Reinventing ourselves, on the other hand, is an ongoing, adventurous journey in life. Like fine wine, each decade should be layered with the richness of our experiences.

Here are some reinvention guidelines to follow:

Guideline Number 1:
Reinvent Yourself Each and Every Decade
Let's face it, the very things you enjoyed in your thirties may not work as you hit forty. Before the age of forty, you may have been busy with your career pursuits, raising a family, dating lots of different guys, or trying to get out of a not-so-perfect relationship. As you approach each decade of your life, take stock of the state of your evolution. Celebrate your successes, eliminate those things that don't fit—like high-maintenance houses or relationships. Continue to evolve, confident that you are adding layers to a rich tapestry of experiences reflected in your inner and outer being.

Guideline Number 2:
Develop Your Secret Power Weapon
My last name is Lyons, so my secret power weapon was a no-brainer: a hefty, 18-karat gold lion's-head ring, complete with diamond eyes and a garnet mouth. I designed this ring when I was in my twenties, and it remains my signature. When I wear it, I feel its power, and experience my own personal strength. People always remember this ring, which helps them remember me.

Your secret power weapon could be a one-of-a-kind designer handbag, or a custom charm bracelet with each charm marking some important personal milestone. Perhaps, like former secretary of state Madeleine Albright, you are a collector of beautiful encrusted pins, and can select the perfect pin to match every occasion.

Guideline Number 3:
Conquer Your Inner Fear of Change
Are you the type who eats the same lunch every day, drives the same route to work, and goes to the same resort year after year with the same group of friends? You may need

to face your fear of changing. Don't disrupt everything all at once. Start small. Instead of going to the same supermarket, try a different one. If you have been thinking about updating your hair style and you admire a stranger's cut, ask who her stylist is. Then go for a consultation.

Guideline Number 4:
What to Do When Life Throws a Curve
Let's face it, life happens just when you're planning other things. The unwelcome change may be personal tragedy, an illness, job woes, or divorce. Take the time to reflect on your reinvention process. This does not mean you have to start over. It just means that you have to figure out how to accommodate this unexpected curve ball so that you can keep evolving.

Guideline Number 5:
Stay Forever Young
The fact that you're aging doesn't mean you have to become old. Become ageless instead. Have a highly developed sense of humor, with the ability to laugh at your own foibles. Be interested in people around you and the world at large. Stay current and keep challenging your mind. Be a good listener, and impart your wisdom and knowledge to others with diplomacy and love. Finally, remember you are one of a kind. There is no one like you of any age in the world. Appreciate your uniqueness, and you will never feel invisible.

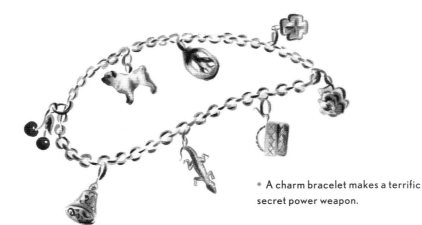

• A charm bracelet makes a terrific secret power weapon.

[Chapter 1]

✦ ✦ ✦

IT'S ABOUT TIME

✳

How are you feeling? Excited? Can't wait to dive in? Or are you looking for an exit or maybe an excuse to put this off for another month, year, or decade? If it's the latter, stay with me for a minute. Let's address the obvious obstacles now. I know how it is. You're already feeling overwhelmed by your busy life, and now you're considering taking on what I like to call Brenda's 30-Day Beauty Camp for Divas. You're asking yourself, "Do I have the time and money for this?" Good question.

The last thing I want you to do is take on something that feels like more stress. Beauty Camp is a totally loving, self-indulgent, fun project. It does involve time and money. These topics are worth chatting about before we get to the details about camp.

Let's talk about money first. This program does not require spending your savings on ball gowns. It does require making a list of needs and allocating funds for them. These may include a long overdue haircut or coloring, some new makeup application tools, and maybe some new, age-appropriate skin products or cosmetics. It's possible that you're using tools and products that are old enough to be considered antiques, and these tools are not giving you the results you want.

You might need to buy some new clothes that will push your wardrobe up a notch or two. The good news is that I'm going to teach you how to shop for diva style on a budget if that suits you. If you've got money in a rainy day account, you may find yourself buying things of better quality than the clothing in your closet. But you'll be investing in things you'll wear for several seasons instead of spending impulsively on trendy items that will be "out" in five minutes. In the past, when you bought clothing, you may have repeated the same mistakes over and over again. Now you'll be shopping for items that you can't wait to wear, things that deserve to take up room in your closet. The truth is, you may end up saving money because your clothing will be well chosen.

I'm not an unlimited-bank-account kind of person and I don't expect you to be, either. In my business, I work with some clients who spend five hundred dollars a year on clothes and others who spend over

twenty thousand. At both financial ends, the women end up with smart wardrobes that suit their needs and play up their diva style.

The next issue, which I think is the biggest one for women, is time. Some parts of the thirty-day program won't demand as much time as others because you're probably stronger in some areas and weaker in others. You may not need to spend extra time on skin care appointments, haircuts, or color because you already pay close attention to these, but maybe your wardrobe needs are greater. You may want to spend more time shopping for key pieces that will make up your diva signature style.

Immersion Therapy

✦ ✦ ✦

So why set this up as a thirty-day program? Why not just give you a list of things to do so you can go out and do it on your own schedule? Well, you can take that route if you like, but here's why I want you to block out a month: You're more likely to have a conversion if you go for immersion. Putting yourself into a unique setting for a while can do a lot to break old habits and create new ones. Before you realize it, you'll find yourself light-years from where you were when you started, as if you went from dowdy to diva!

Think about this. If you wanted to get better at cooking, you could take a cooking class twice a month in the evening and learn a few new

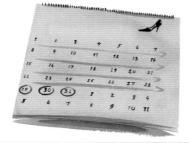

dishes to try out on your family or friends. Now think about what it would be like to have the cooking instructor with you in your pantry, helping you reorganize for greater efficiency, telling you which dried herbs to banish forever, and how to stock your shelves so you can whip up a gorgeous meal for eight at a moment's notice. Since you have to eat every day, this kind of immersion would surely leave you with lasting new habits that you could use immediately.

We're going to do the same thing with something else you do every day—getting dressed. You're going to get into your closets and shelves and find out what's gone bad, and which fresh things to bring in so you can dress for any occasion in minutes. That's worth carving out time for. You can tell your family, your friends, and your coworkers, or make it your little secret. Just stay with me for thirty days. If you have to leave camp because of some unexpected, demanding activities, just come back as soon as you can. The Diva Advisors will be here waiting for you, and so will I.

There's a lot more to you than you may think. Beyond your job, kids, grandkids, husband, extended family, and your health concerns, there's a seed inside of you. It holds the DNA of your diva. You need to separate yourself from day-to-day concerns so you can get to that place of knowingness, assuredness, and wholeness that lives within. To find it, you will need to set aside some time for camp activities. It's hard to find that gushing well of knowledge when you're too darn busy. So if you hear a sentence that starts, "Honey, could you just . . ." be prepared to say no. Give your kids, lover, and friends a heads-up that you're not to be counted on for anything new over the next thirty days. That's doable, isn't it?

You'll be more engaged and your results will be more profound if you really focus on yourself and your needs. Therefore, this will not be the month when you volunteer to head up a fundraising drive for your local hospital. This is also not the time to do any of the following:

✦ Come up with plans to remodel the kitchen

✦ Plan a family reunion

✦ Research colleges for your kid

✦ Cochair the annual Cattle Baron's Ball to raise money for cancer research

✦ Start writing your dissertation

✦ Begin a new diet

✦ Host your book group

✦ Organize your husband's office

✦ Organize your office

✦ Be the wedding planner for your best friend

✦ Sew matching quilts for the new twins in the family

✦ Work on your relationship with your significant other

✦ Begin or end an affair

✦ _____.

(Add your own here.)

The Dowdy Quiz

✦ ✦ ✦

Let's address what I hope is the last obstacle—that tiny bit of doubt you have about whether or not you even need to update your look. You might be a diva already!

I've created a quiz for you to take that will help you see where you are on the scale of dowdy to diva. Circle the answer that best sums up your current state of mind and affairs.

1. You get invited to opening night of the film festival and, because you know the organizer, you will get to sit at the same table as the visiting movie stars. You reply

a. "Yes, I'm there!" and go to your closet to pull out the perfect outfit.

b. "Can I get back to you?" Then you run out of the house to do some panic shopping.

c. "Gosh, I'd go, but *CSI* is on tonight and I don't have TiVo." You *do* have TiVo. You *don't* have party clothes.

d. "I don't do parties." You stay home with the remote and a box of chocolates because the thought of finding something to wear to such an event is paralyzing.

2. Your jewelry stash is made up of

a. A mix of good costume jewelry plus some of the real stuff.

b. A tangled mess of gold chains that your husband buys you every year for your birthday.

c. Macaroni necklaces your kids made you.

d. Jewelry? What jewelry?

3. You spend money on clothes. When it comes to the accessories to go with them, you

a. Refuse to go home without the shoes, handbag, and jewelry that will make your outfit pop.

b. Have confidence the jewelry you have at home will be good enough.

c. Say "I've spent my quota, I'll think about the accessories later."

d. Think the salesperson is just trying to mess with you when she makes accessory suggestions.

4. The last time you put a total look together—the dress, makeup, hair, and accessories—was

a. Yesterday.

b. Last week.

c. Last year.

d. The day you got married (the first time).

5. The last time you really felt attractive was

a. Yesterday while driving car pool.

b. Last week when you got dressed up for girls' night out.

c. Last year when you went to your cousin's wedding.

d. The day you got married.

6. The last time you went shopping for yourself was

a. Last month — just for fun.

b. Last year when your sister was visiting from Canada.

c. Three years ago at an outlet mall.

d. Fifteen years ago when the divorce was final.

7. The last time you got fitted for a bra was

a. Six months ago.

b. Last year.

c. Ten years ago.

d. When you were twelve.

8. The last time you gave your hair a style adjustment was

a. Six months ago.

b. In 2003.

c. In 1999.

d. In 1985.

9. Your makeup look is

a. Created by using five or more products.

b. Lipstick if you're going out.

c. Mascara and concealer, once in a while.

d. *Au naturel* — you don't wear makeup.

10. If someone suggests you try something on in a color you've never worn, you

a. Are excited to see if this new color will look good on you.

b. Pull out the color palette you had done twenty years ago. If the color isn't among your swatches, you say, "No, I can't wear that."

c. Barely hide your irritation as you sneer, "I don't think so."

d. Walk away because it isn't black.

11. You've been wearing the same lipstick shade since

a. Christmas.

b. Last summer.

c. The babies were in diapers.

d. Kennedy was president.

12. When it comes to fit, you

a. Buy whatever size is the most flattering and fine-tune the fit with an alterations person.

b. Squeeze into a size 12 no matter how it looks.

c. Buy things that are loose, so fit doesn't matter that much anyway.

d. Buy something in the wrong size, think you can fix it, but never do.

13. Over the years your body has shifted its weight into different parts. You're fully aware of this and you

a. Have stopped shopping in the junior departments and happily shop in the missy departments.

b. Shop in catalogues geared to "women of a certain age."

c. Wear the same two things over and over. You're sure you'll get back to that shape you were fifteen years ago, and when you do, you'll wear all those things you loved back then.

d. Refuse to go shopping and have resorted to wearing tentlike outfits with no body definition to them.

14. The last time someone said, "Wow, you look great!" was

a. Yesterday.

b. Last week.

c. Last year.

d. Sometime in 1985.

15. You get your fashion and beauty advice from

a. Your trusted friend, who once worked for Vera Wang.

b. Your husband.

c. The Sunday newspaper supplement ads, which suggest you buy this season's must-have skirt.

d. Back issues of *Good Housekeeping* magazine that you read in the doctor's waiting room.

If most of your answers were "a":

You've been visiting makeup counters, you are aware of fashion trends, and maybe dabble in them. Camp for you will be fun and exciting because you're already enjoying fashion and beauty, and this program will multiply that joy tenfold. It's possible that on a scale from 1 to 10 — 10 being diva signature style — you're somewhere between a 4 and an 8. I'm guessing that if you apply the tricks and tips you'll learn in camp and couple them with your existing efforts, you'll have diva style perfected in no time. While in camp, you'll be able to figure out what you're already doing right and gain the knowledge and experience necessary to take your look to new confident heights.

If most of your answers were "b":

You're making an effort. You may not trust a lot of people. Or maybe you just haven't found the right people to supply you with information that you feel comfortable adapting to your own look. You'll benefit from this step-by-step program because you're in good hands. Your time and money will be well spent and you'll see dramatic results once you've devoted some extra hours this month to improving your skill with clothes and makeup.

If most of your answers were "c":

Self-neglect has taken its toll. When you don't like how you look, you hold yourself back from fully participating in the opportunities that come your way. You've suffered from "blahtosis" long enough! Maybe there hasn't been much time or space for experimentation with your personal appearance, or maybe lethargy is holding you back. Not to worry. We'll wake up your senses once you get to camp. By saying yes to yourself and Beauty Camp, you're going to be saying yes to lots of things. When you look good, you feel good. Believe it or not, once you've been to Beauty Camp, life gets easier in every way!

If most of your answers were "d":

Your makeover is going to be off the charts. It will be like turning a falling-down barn into an art museum, or a barren hill into a robust vineyard. Everyone's going to be convinced you're having an affair or just got off a sabbatical in the Caribbean. There's no way but up for you! Once you've completed this program, you'll be one of those women who will have everyone guessing. They'll be wondering, Did she lose ten pounds? Has she met someone? You'll want to be vigilant about carving time out for yourself. Use every time-saving tip I give you. You may not have much in your closet to work with, so you'll want to spend lots of time in dressing rooms and maybe even just browsing through stores to train your eyes to recognize what you love.

An Invitation

✦ ✦ ✦

I invite you to Brenda's 30-Day Beauty Camp for Divas. You're welcome just as you are. Regardless of your background or knowledge of style and beauty, you have every chance of being successful in this program. Divas come in all shapes and sizes and include all nationalities. Shy or outgoing, you'll fit right in.

Get a buddy to go through this process with you if you like. You know how much fun it is to go to camp with a pal. Together you can help each other through the exercises and the scavenger hunts for great diva pieces. You can also support each other as you get ready to go on your dates.

I'm here for you. I'll hold your hand. Diva Advisors Sunny and Gary Yates are here for you too. Today they're going to help you prepare for success with their tips for sticking to this program. This makeover project might seem like a lot, but step-by-step we'll get there. You have everything to gain and you're going to have so much fun! I'll see you at camp orientation!

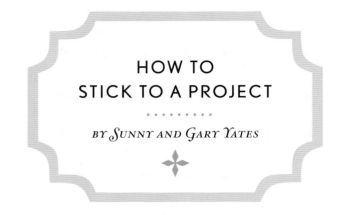

HOW TO STICK TO A PROJECT

. . . .

BY SUNNY AND GARY YATES

✦

Diva Advisors Sunny and Gary Yates founded Effective Environments, a national consulting firm, in 1994. The Yateses have developed a way of thinking and working that boosts effectiveness. They've created steps to ensure your success at Beauty Camp.

To begin, remember that Beauty Camp is about making yourself a priority and expressing yourself as the diva you know yourself to be. Here are eight tips to help you along:

1. Make *you* your number one priority. This may be the first time you've done this. Beware of the ways you may unconsciously sabotage yourself—by thinking, for example, "I'll meet my needs when everyone else has been taken care of."

2. Create a vision of your successful participation in Beauty Camp and the difference it will make in your life. Capture it in words or pictures and keep it where you will see it every day. If you like, put together a collage. Make your vision so enticing that no obstacles will get in your way. Your vision will remind you, when the going gets tough, of why you're doing this.

3. Garner support from everyone around you. Promises we make only to ourselves are easier to break than the ones we share openly with others. For example, say to your family, "I'm committed to completing these assignments for camp this week. Will you be in charge of dinner, make your own lunches, and minimize the interruptions?" Report back on your successes, and acknowledge everyone's contributions!

4. Create your master plan for Beauty Camp. Break the project into bite-size pieces. It's easier to fit them into a busy schedule, and it's hugely motivating to check things off quickly! Each week make a list of everything you intend to do as part of Beauty Camp. Then put a date beside every task. Be realistic and *tell the truth* about when you will do each one.

5. Focus on specific outcomes. Sometimes, results are not dependent on the time we put into them. Planning to devote two hours to a project may not be an effective strategy because (a) you may not have an easy time finding a two-hour block of time, (b) you may discover you don't actually *need* two hours in order to make it happen, and (c) without the clear focus on an outcome, devoting two hours may not produce what you want. Be sure you have clear, specific outcomes in mind, and be open to multiple ways of achieving them.

6. Set boundaries. Put a sign on the door saying, "Not available except in an emergency until 7:00 p.m." Resist the urge to answer every phone call or every e-mail until a specified future time. Consciously put yourself first.

7. Use an anchor. Find a talisman, photo, quote, amulet, or another small physical reminder of the project and why you are doing it. A butterfly pin symbolizing transformation may remind you 24/7 of your commitment to yourself and keep you motivated.

8. Above all, mark your accomplishments! Celebrate every achievement. Give yourself a pat on the back, or a special treat. If you go off track, *forgive yourself.* All is not lost. The game isn't over until you quit. Create a new plan and begin again.

+ ✦ +

Chapter 2

WELCOME TO BRENDA'S 30-DAY BEAUTY CAMP

✻

Yay! You made the decision to come to camp! You're going to love it here. Before you begin this week's activities, I want to let you know all about camp and how to get the most out of it. There are some things to shop for, items to clear off your calendar, and some last-minute preparations before we get started. Did I tell you who else is here? Experts in beauty, clothing style, hair, makeup, and emergency fashion triage have flown in to make guest appearances. They'll be assisting you as you move your look from whatever level of dowdy you might feel you're in to diva all the way.

You're doing Beauty Camp from right where you are. That's convenient. No bags to pack, long airplane rides, or layovers in foreign countries. You're operating from home! Here are some ground rules.

Since you're at home, you need to put yourself in a time-out. That's right. You're in a time-out for the next four weeks. So take care of any last-minute arrangements for getting as much of a vacation from the demands of everyday life as you can. If you're self-employed, put a message on your business line that says you're out until the Tuesday after next or longer. If work is something you drive to, take some of those personal days or vacation days you've been saving up, and devote them to Beauty Camp. Put a message on your home phone that says you'll be away. Do the same with your e-mail.

Get it in your head and on your calendar that your time is booked—for you. If you're not good at this, call a couple of friends over to help you do a scheduling intervention. Turn your calendar or your appointment book over to them and ask them to rearrange your days so you have more time for yourself. This works; I do it myself. And then train your friends and your family members to leave you alone. The only interruptions that you'll acknowledge are policemen at the door and spurting blood, in which case you will make the 911 phone call. Other than that, you're off limits. You're at camp.

There are some supplies to shop for. You can find most of the listed items at a stationery store, office supply store, or drug store. Other items can be picked up at a store that specializes in either closet organizers or bath items. Do your shopping and then meet me back here for orientation.

Here's what you'll need:

✦ Diva journal. This is a diary for you to write about your adventures at Beauty Camp. Alternatively, you could devote a section of a three-ring binder to your private thoughts, a-ha moments, and comments along the way. Make the cover appealing so you look forward to writing in it. You can put a picture that you love in the front sleeve of your three-ring binder if that's what you will use.

✦ Three-ring binder, section dividers, and plastic sheet protectors

✦ Stack of fashion magazines and/or catalogues

✦ Glue stick and black paper close to card stock weight

✦ Presentation book (look at Itoya's Web site, www.itoya.com, for examples)

✦ Heavy-duty trash bags (for bagging up dowdy clothes that are making an exit from your life)

✦ Hangers in one color and style to replace the mismatched hangers in your closet

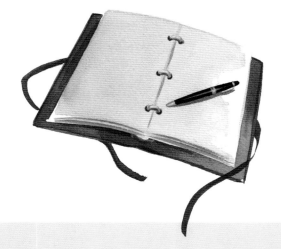

Camp Orientation

+ + +

I've put the steps of your dowdy-to-diva transformation into a four-week time frame. Feel free to expand that time frame as needed. If you need two weeks to complete the assignments in Week Two, take them. Some parts of camp might consume more of your energy than others.

Week One can be conducted in your jammies as you begin to pull together the elements of your diva style. The exercises we'll do involve ripping pages out of magazines and searching your home for style clues. You'll be identifying your ruts and generally paying attention to what resonates for you so you can dress for who you are now. You'll put your a-ha's into your diva journal.

In Week Two you'll spend most of the time at home in your closet—taking hikes through your wardrobe, swimming through your underwear drawer, going on a scavenger hunt for the really cool diva pieces you already own, and bringing them front and center so you can appreciate and wear them.

In Week Three, you'll be leaving the house for the field trip part of Beauty Camp—shopping and collecting possible pieces for three specific outfits. The outfits will be designed for the three dates, which I'll discuss in a moment. Each date, and therefore each outfit, will focus on a different aspect of your lifestyle, ranging from dressy to casual. You might decide to do some of your shopping with a friend as you explore new stores.

In Week Four you'll be out and about getting beauty treatments as required. You'll need to make some appointments in advance. Even before that, you'll want to gather recommendations for hair and makeup professionals. Review chapters 12 and 13 on hair and makeup this week. There are many suggestions to help you decide which types of professionals you want to see. Diva Advisor Felicia Gelardi will persuade you to set up some skin care appointments before Week Four (see page 180). That's the week when you'll also be putting the final touches of your diva look together so you'll be fully prepared for your three dates. You'll learn how to accept the inevitable compliments, too. And we'll make sure you know how to look good in the photos that the paparazzi (or your kids) will be taking of you to mark your transformation.

• You'll be spending Week One in your jammies.

Appearing throughout camp will be our expert Diva Advisors, who are interested in supporting your efforts. There will also be seasoned divas, who will share their tips for style and beauty in sidebars called Diva Sense. You'll also get to meet a few divas up close and personal. They will let you into their closets and their heads in Diva Spotlights.

Every week there will be specific exercises and tasks to accomplish. There will also be breaks—time to go off on your own. At the end of each chapter is a beauty soak, a relaxing activity that will let you soak in what you've been learning while keeping you immersed in the healing quality of beauty. This is a creative process, and you'll need time to assimilate everything. Plan for good rest and good meals so you can think clearly and be mentally strong.

After you learn about your style preferences and create your own unique look at Beauty Camp, you'll test those skills by going on those three dates, which I mentioned earlier. Start deciding what those dates will be. I suggest you make Date One an evening social event, such as a party, the theater, opera, or dinner at a nice restaurant and a movie. Choose whatever is at the formal end of your social life. Stretch

yourself! It could also be a festive event like a wedding, a high school reunion, or an anniversary party. Can you imagine walking into that gourmet restaurant and meeting friends who haven't seen you since you started Beauty Camp? It's going to be great!

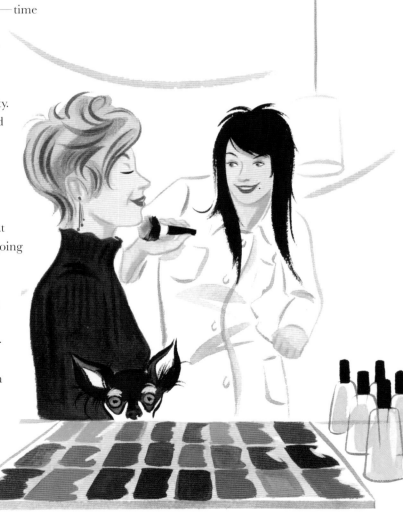

• By Week Four you'll be ready for a makeup update.

Date Two is an event that would fall into the daytime weekend category—a birthday lunch with friends, a visit to a museum, a religious event, or even a day of shopping. Once and for all, you will learn how to put together a casual outfit that has style and looks polished.

Date Three is an event at your home, an intimate dinner party or cocktails and hors d'oeuvres for you and friends, or a private experience for just you and your honey. Why not stretch yourself in terms of where you will go to show off your new look? Maybe you've put off attending some of the cool things you've been reading about in the entertainment section of your newspaper. How about picking one of those things for one of your dates? Ask friends who are in the know where the newest hot spots are. Go for an experience, and make it special. Splurge on an elegant dinner out at a trendy new restaurant. You won't have to worry about what you're going to wear. By the time you finish camp, you'll know what's appropriate.

After you've gone on your three dates, your chariot won't turn into a pumpkin. I'm going to leave you with ways to carry on in true diva style. You'll learn more about that in the last chapter, Diva Forever, where we reflect on your accomplishments and make plans for the future.

There. I think it's all been covered, except the dress code. I'm not going to make you wear uniform camp T-shirts in that shade of orange that flatters 1 percent of the population. No, you have only one rule for what you wear to camp each day, and it's this: wear what you love. If you stay in your jammies for the first week, as I promised you could, then make them your favorite jammies. If you have a silk nightgown and matching robe that you've put away for a special day, that day has arrived. Nothing is too good or too precious to wear to camp.

Ready? Got your shopping done? You've picked out your camp uniform? Okay, then. Get ready for Week One of beauty camp!

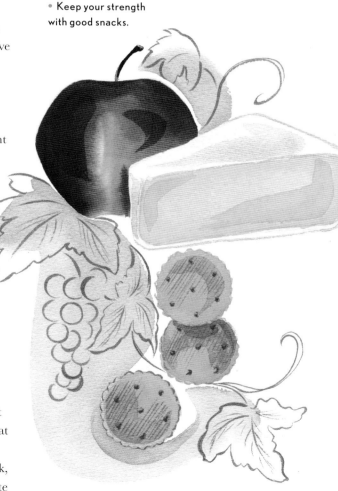

• Keep your strength with good snacks.

WEEK ONE

Chapter 3 • **RUTS**

PAGE 30

Chapter 4 • **RESONANCE**

PAGE 45

Chapter 5 • **COLOR YOUR WORLD**

PAGE 49

Chapter 6 • **DEFINING YOUR DIVA STYLE**

PAGE 61

Chapter 7 • **FIT FOR A DIVA**

PAGE 78

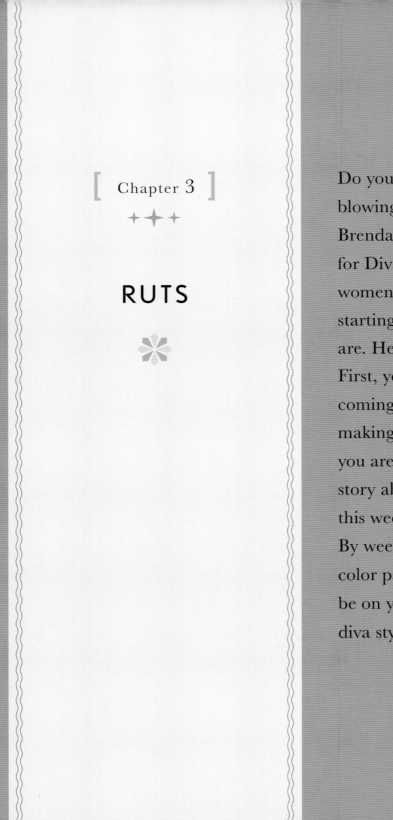

[Chapter 3]

✦ ✦ ✦

RUTS

Do you hear that? The whistle is blowing, signaling the first day of Brenda's 30-Day Beauty Camp for Divas. Welcome! You're joining women all over the world who are starting diva camp today, just as you are. Here's the schedule for the week: First, you'll set the dates for your coming-out events, where you'll be making your entrance as the diva you are. Later on today, you'll hear a story about Susan that will introduce this week's focus: ruts and resonance. By week's end, you'll have created a color palette that you love, and you'll be on your way to defining your true diva style.

You're also going to participate in beauty soak activities, which immerse you in the nourishing qualities of beauty. Feel free to go beyond my suggestions and come up with some of your own ideas. By completing a beauty soak each week, you'll get into the habit of taking care of yourself and renewing your diva spirit. Ready? Set? Let's go!

Diva Dates

✦ ✦ ✦

To begin, I'd like you to work out the details of your coming-out dates roughly a month from now. Let's start with your dressy date: Is there a play you've been wanting to see? Are you interested in attending the opera or a ballet? If you are from a small town or a farming area, a big night out may be going to a church dinner. That will do. You don't need to travel five hours to the big city in order to have fun. But then again, if that's something you've been thinking about, this is the time to do it! You're getting out of your old routines, so shake things up. Consider doing one of the things you've put off for "someday." Someday is here.

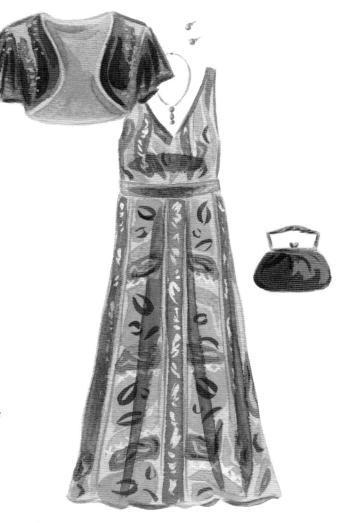

• Dressy. A flirty print dress with a shrug is perfect for a festive get-together.

•• Dressy Date ••

Jot down as many details as you can about your dressy date. What arrangements can you make this week? Commit! Don't worry about the last item, your outfit. We'll get to that later.

•• Dressy Date Details ••

Date activity:

Scheduled for (time and date):

Place:

People involved:

Phone calls to make (reservations, tickets, etc.):

Other action steps to take:

Support people to schedule (babysitters, car rental, etc.):

Hair, makeup, or grooming appointments to make:

Outfit (to be determined):

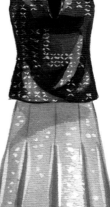

• Dressy. Luxurious fabrics in simple shapes make for festive party attire.

• Dressy. Pair a dressy top with a special skirt for a special date.

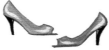

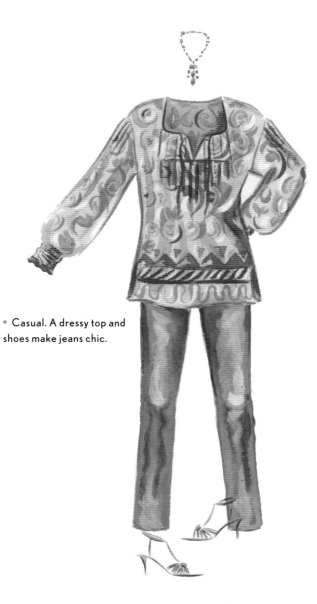

• Casual. A dressy top and shoes make jeans chic.

•• Casual Date ••

Now, what casual date do you plan to go on? It could be a birthday luncheon for a friend, or a Saturday matinee performance of a one-woman show. You could go to a museum for the day and meet a friend later for dinner. If you need to make reservations or call someone and invite them to this event, do it this week. Get the ball rolling. Fill in the details that you know.

•• Casual Date Details ••

Date activity:
....

Scheduled for (time and date):
....

Place:
....

People involved:
....

Phone calls to make (reservations, tickets, etc.):
....

....

Other action steps to take:
....

....

Support people to schedule (babysitters, car rental, etc.):
....

....

Hair, makeup, or grooming appointments to make:
....

....

Outfit (to be determined):
....

....

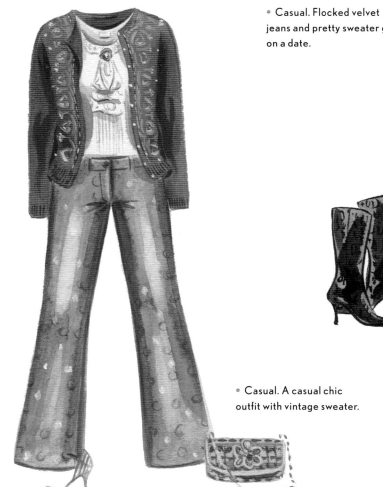

• Casual. Flocked velvet
jeans and pretty sweater go
on a date.

• Casual. A casual chic
outfit with vintage sweater.

·· At Home Date ··

Now, the last date is something you'll be doing from home. You decide whether it will be a dinner party, a cocktail party, or an intimate date with your sweetheart. This is going to be grown-up time. You're not planning a grandchild's birthday party or overseeing your daughter's graduation party. Regardless of whether it's a private party for two or a party for six or more, you'll be the belle of the ball, and I'll show you how.

To give you more confidence in the arena of home entertaining, I've brought in Diva Advisor Cheryl Simmons. Cheryl has been a professional party planner for thirty years. She plans events of all sizes with a range of budgets, and she's agreed to help you prepare for your at-home event.

Although you may be planning some of this event during the coming month, take your best shot at filling in the details of your at-home date. And remember, if you think you need to remodel the bathroom in order to have friends over, then alter the plan. Plan a picnic at a nearby park or go for something intimate with someone who doesn't mind using the bathroom just the way it is.

·· At-Home Date Details ··

Date activity:
....

Scheduled for (time and date):
....

Place:
....

People involved:
....

....

Other action steps to take:
....

....

Support people to schedule (caterer, house cleaner, etc.):
....

....

Hair, makeup, or grooming appointments to make:
....

....

Outfit (to be determined):
....

....

• At home. Simple shapes in elegant colors—white and gold—are great for hostessing.

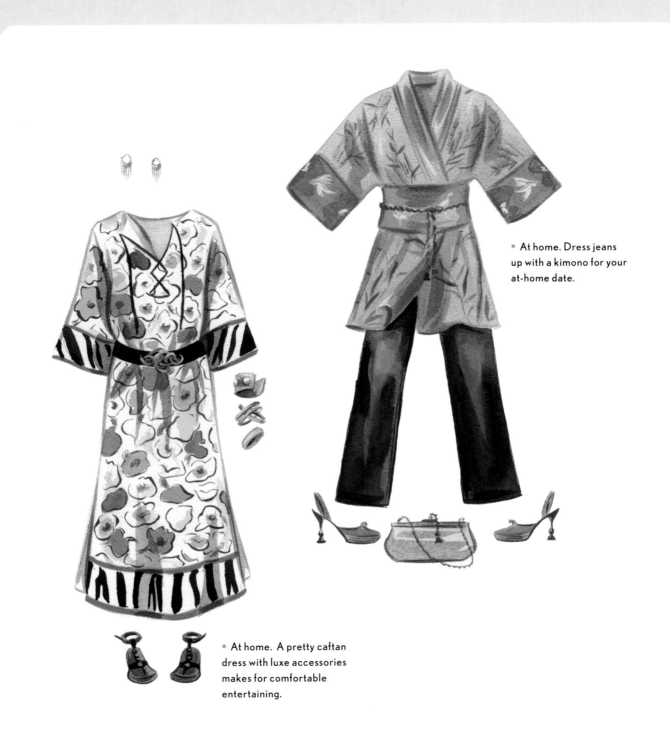

• At home. Dress jeans up with a kimono for your at-home date.

• At home. A pretty caftan dress with luxe accessories makes for comfortable entertaining.

HOW TO THROW A SUCCESSFUL PARTY

BY CHERYL SIMMONS

The four basic elements of a great event are an intriguing invitation, an inviting opener, a pleasing ambience, and a memorable favor or going-home gift. If you're planning an intimate party with just your sweetheart, you may be the party favor!

1. The invitation is the first thing your guests see. It needs to grab them and give them enough info to titillate but not so much that you give it all away. A good stationery store will have cute ready-made invitations. If you're inviting friends over for popcorn and movies, create an oversized ticket stub as an invitation with all the pertinent information on it. If it's a sexy date you're planning, you could take Scrabble letter tiles, spell out *Romance*, and mail it to your lover with the time and place of your date.

2. When your guests move into your environment, you want them to experience a wow factor. It could be you greeting them with a smile and a generous hello, or it could be a white-gloved butler. Or you can hire your kids or friends and instruct them to serve pretty cocktail party drinks as soon as guests arrive.

3. Ambience is as easy as having music playing, especially if it relates to the theme of the party. A log can be burning in the fireplace. Candlelight is always inviting.

4. If you have a dinner party, the only thing people will remember is whether you served great desserts. The last thing they eat is what they'll talk about. That and the party favors. If the party has a theme, connect the favors with it.

Here are three easy party ideas.

1. Plan a picnic at home for two. Get a blanket and candles and put together a basket. If it's your style, fill it with china, real crystal glasses, pâté and cheeses, crackers, and a chilled bottle of Dom Perignon. Or use paper plates and sparkling cider. The blanket could be cashmere or a traditional camping blanket. Don't use hot food: get food from a deli counter. Have pillows around; you might need them for later.

2. For a night-at-the-movies party, rent DVDs that you know your friends will appreciate. It could be anything from a Jim Carrey comedy to the classic *Casablanca*. Purchase candies that you'd find at a movie theater and arrange them in a basket.

3. You can plan a party with an Asian theme. Buy inexpensive Asian dinnerware, such as sake cups and rice bowls. Wrap up pretty chopsticks with ribbon. You can even hire a sushi chef. Order fortune cookies, but write your own fortunes.

Regardless of what type of party you're having, a relaxed hostess is a must, and that means you. Have everything in place the night before. The day of the event, your only job is to be beautiful.

Meet Susan

✦ ✦ ✦

Susan is in her mid-forties, married, and living in the San Francisco Bay Area. An intelligent woman with a sharp wit, she's been a twenty-year fan of a popular Bay Area radio call-in show. She introduced herself to the host, Ron, years ago via e-mail, as callers are invited to do. She and Ron liked to debate issues respectfully, but they'd never met in person. When she heard that a nationally known host of a popular cooking program from the Food Network channel was coming to the show, she shot off an e-mail asking Ron if she could be in the studio during the interview. The guest was one of her cooking heroes.

Permission was granted, and, the day of the interview, she got dressed in her uniform: She wore an ivory cashmere twin sweater set, black slacks, sensible black shoes, her good jewelry—a gold pendant and matching earrings from Tiffany's—and her plain black handbag with a shoulder strap. When Susan arrived, she was introduced to the staff, the host, and the guest, who paid as much attention to her as the palm tree in the corner of the studio. "That's okay," she thought, "I'm just here to watch. I'll just be a mouse in the corner." She pulled up a studio chair as the interview was about to begin. That's when Ron looked over at her and confessed, "You know, Susan, I know nothing about cooking and you're a big fan of this guy's show. You should be doing this interview, not me. What do you say? Are you game?"

"Okay" slipped out of her mouth, and before she could reconsider, a headset appeared and she was seated opposite the cooking star. The host announced the change of plans on air, saying this would be the "Susan hour."

Susan's in the software business and works from her home office. She had never been to a radio studio before or done anything as on-the-spot as this interview. She was nervous, but when she listened to the tape afterward, she heard what everyone else in the Bay Area heard—a professional interview with smart, engaging questions and great entertainment throughout the hour. I heard the tape. You'd think she'd been a radio personality her whole life. I wanted to hear more interviews by her!

On her drive home from the radio station that day, Susan had a lot swimming around in her mind. She was on such a high. She realized that this experience, completely spontaneous and unexpected, had been the most fun she'd had in years. She saw a part of herself that wasn't being expressed in her proper and safe conservative image. What had been so comfortable to her for years—her nice sweater set, gold jewelry, and black pants—was suddenly ill-fitting. She wanted to look the way she felt during that interview: sassy, bold, and visible. There was nothing wrong with what she'd been wearing. It just wasn't her anymore. She called me shortly after this event and told me about her epiphany. She wanted her outside to match this newly discovered inside part of her.

We got right to it, and quickly identified a few ruts. Susan had gotten in the habit of buying jewelry from one place only — Tiffany's — all of it in gold and in matching sets. In fact, almost everything she bought was either in sets or in duplicates — the same sweater set in every color, the same shoe in three colors, the same handbag in four colors. It added up to "predict-able." Nice enough, but ordinary, which is not Susan!

In short order, we traded in most of the sweater sets for tops in lively colorful prints and in fabrics with interesting, begging-to-be-touched textures. We found pants that were more sexy than the ones she'd been wearing. Instead of wearing two neutral colors at one time, she wore three colors or more, and some of them were even bright. She didn't stop wearing the gold Tiffany jewelry altogether, but we did buy good costume pieces and mixed them in with the precious jewelry. We added hits of color in unexpected places, like handbags or novelty jackets. No longer was she living in a beige and black world. Now she had color and energy in her wardrobe! Her appearance matched her exuberance for life. Now she's an everyday diva— every day.

I'm thinking maybe you've been living smaller than you are. Maybe you've got a few ruts yourself. Let's get you out of them so you can enjoy a look that's more you, just as Susan did. You may express different qualities than Susan, but that personal connection to clothes can be yours soon.

Excavating Ruts

✦ ✦ ✦

Being in a fashion rut is a lot like being in a bad relationship. Before we find our way out of one, we often spend years feeling stuck, going through the motions while never feeling satisfied or happy. We ignore our needs and make ourselves small enough to fit into a tight box, expressing nothing of our true passion. Been there? Contrast the feelings of being in a bad relationship to the exhilaration and youthfulness you feel when you fall in love. You know that glow that people have when they're in love? They look ten years younger, and ten pounds thinner. They radiate lusciousness. That's the kind of glow you're going to be wearing when you say "buh-bye" to your fashion ruts and find clothes you love that love you back. Today is the day to face what's *not* working, to name it so you can have it in your rearview mirror four weeks from now.

DIVA SENSE

"I went to my closet one day, opened the door, and saw dress after dress in sweet floral prints. They had been my trademark for years. Suddenly I thought, I need a black leather jacket by tomorrow or I'll scream. I was so done with the floral prints. I boxed them all up, sent them to my sister, and then went out and bought that leather jacket. I felt instantly relieved. Finally, I was comfortable inside my own skin."

Jill

When you admit your ruts, you will move toward your diva style more easily and quickly. If you "break up" with your old look today and stop making excuses, you may have a new look by next Tuesday!

Put on your detective hat and poke around your house with your journal and a pen. I'll tell you about some places where ruts like to hang out: Start by checking out your contributions to the dirty clothes hamper or the hamper that holds whatever is headed for the cleaners. Are all your things black? That's a clue that you may be in a color(less) rut.

Open your makeup drawer. Was everything in there purchased before the new millennium? Is the packaging still on the eye shadows, and are the lipsticks in their little boxes? You could be in a makeup rut.

Look inside your closet. When you go to pull something off the shelf, does a pile of stuff fall down, stuff you forgot you even had? Do you slide your arm in to pull out something on a hanger and fear that you won't be able to get your arm back out because things are so jammed in there? Living with too much clutter could be your rut. You could be missing key diva pieces in there because they are being crushed to death.

Go through your jewelry stash. Do you see viable pieces there, or is it mostly macaroni necklaces and broken seashell bracelets?

Now go to your coat closet. Got some showstoppers there or drab hand-me-downs? Look at your shoes. Are they looking pretty shabby? Can you see why the diva hasn't had a chance to surface? She's buried in an avalanche of neglect and clutter!

If you want a cheat sheet, here are some ruts that people have shared with me:

+ "Buying clothes, but never shopping for the accessories that finish the outfit, so the clothes go unworn."

+ "Buying clothes that are fixer uppers, usually on sale (they just need to be redesigned to fit me right). Only I never get around to fixing them up. In fact, the tags are still hanging on them."

+ "Being stuck in a decade when I was really cool—like high school, when I wore white lipstick, go-go boots, and Farrah Fawcett hair."

+ "Using the same handbag year after year, even when it's scuffed and the handle is hanging by a thread."

+ "Wearing basic everything—clothes and accessories—but not ever enjoying any personal expression in my outfits."

+ "Relying on one clothing piece (jeans!) to wear to everything in life."

+ "Going from the gym to the store to picking up the kids to making dinner, all in my gym clothes."

+ "Going without makeup for the last fifteen years, even when I suspected a little something on my face would feel and look better."

"I love beautiful clothes. I especially love designers like Yohji Yamamoto. I have great clothes, but I used to bring the same handbag everywhere — a Dooney and Bourke black bag that I got at a secondhand store. Even my friends nagged me about it. I was nervous about bags, felt I didn't understand them. But then I went on a shopping trip and focused just on handbags. I bought a few — some for work, some for evening, some for fun. Now I enjoy changing them according to my outfits and my mood. I just had to get over my fear and focus on fixing that one thing about my wardrobe."

Ann

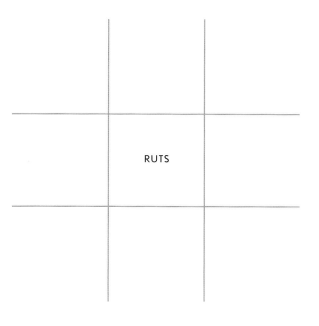

You're going to list some of your ruts on a tic-tac-toe grid. You remember those, right—the game with Xs and Os that you might have played with your siblings on long car trips? Use the grid on this page or make a tic-tac-toe grid on a big piece of paper right now. In the center of it write the word "ruts." Then in the eight remaining boxes, where you'd have put an X or an O, write out the key ruts that you'd like to be moving away from for good.

Keep this list with your other style notes and exercises. Thirty days from now, you'll look back on this grid you've made today, and I predict you'll have worked through many, if not all, of these ruts. You will have replaced old bad habits with new strategies for pleasing yourself. Where will you find those new strategies? You're going to begin capturing them in your resonance book, which contains the vision for everything you *do* want. You'll find out more about resonance books in the next chapter.

DIVA SENSE

"My biggest rut is that I buy something that is too much like what I already own. I have several brown sweaters and I always look the same regardless of which one I wear."

Lynn

Now, with your ruts in mind, I want you to start considering what might take their place. This exercise is called Moving Away From and Moving Toward. In your diva journal, write "Moving Away From" on the left-hand side of the page, and "Moving Toward" on the right-hand side. For everything that you want to move away from (no date clothes, too many choices, not enough choices, clothes that don't fit), identify what you want to move toward (date clothes, fewer but better choices, more variety, clothes that fit now).

Living with ruts is often an unconscious choice. Here in Beauty Camp, you're going to be making conscious decisions every day. You're going to stay awake to your needs and desires for a full thirty days. No more accepting the unacceptable. No more excuses. Everything you wear and everything you do to your face, your hair, and your body will be for a good reason: that's the way you really want it.

DIVA SENSE

"I'd like to move away from resenting my post-menopausal shape and move toward accepting it and appreciating it.

I'd like to move away from wearing boring everyday clothes to wearing clothes I enjoy.

I'd like to move away from uncreative outfits to creative ones.

I'd like to move away from an unfocused look to a pulled-together look.

I'd like to move away from settling for pants I don't like because they fit, and move toward wearing great-looking and -fitting pants.

I'd like to move away from looking in my closet and thinking 'Yuck,' and get closer to looking in my closet and thinking 'Yes!'

I'd like to move away from a scattershot approach to clothes buying and move toward a more cohesive approach.

I'd like to move away from 'It's okay to be invisible' and toward being happily visible." *Marilyn*

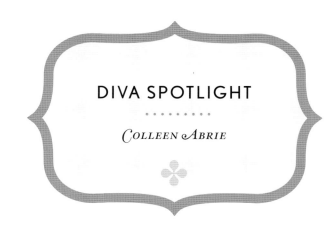

DIVA SPOTLIGHT

·········

Colleen Abrie

For the past twenty-six years, I've been working with hair and makeup for guys and gals. I especially love styling photo shoots, doing hair color and makeup updates, and providing commentary on celebrity hairstyles for various publications. I love luxuriating. It can be visual beauty of any kind, music, food, or laughter. I have eighteen skirts in my closet. Yes, they all fit, and I wear them all.

What colors do you wear to flatter your natural coloring?

Since I am aging, my colors are a little softer and not as vivid as when I was younger. I wear skin tone shades instead of white. They are much kinder to my skin after I've had too many margaritas. I wear rose tones to project sweetness and attract empathy. People feel for you when you wear these shades, so if you need nurturing, wear them and the world will nurture you! Berry is my favorite. It's not red or violet, but right in between, and luscious like a slice of berry pie. I wear violet, usually deeper tones, when I want to project mystery and keep the riffraff at arm's length. I have fallen in love with deep espresso brown for two reasons: it's softer than black, and it looks to-die-for with skin tones, rose tones, berries, violets, reds, denim, blues, greens — everything.

How do you flatter your assets?

I stick to hourglass silhouettes, since that is my figure type. I like fabrics that drape and feel good. A-line skirts and full-leg trousers are my secret weapons. I have core wardrobe pieces that are related to my hair and eye colors. They go with anything I buy, and make me look really pulled together without my thinking about it.

Name a key diva piece.

Lipstick. How could you even think you were a diva and leave the house without lip color? Heck, it's still on my lips when I go to bed.

What are your accessory must-haves?

I can never have too many necklaces. They change my look and style statement instantly.

An old favorite that you still wear?

My pink-and-olive tie-dyed T-shirt. I can't give it away yet. Also, my pointy-toed black high heels will always have a place in my evening wear.

Name something you splurged on and never looked back.

My shearling jacket, which I bought five years ago. I've already worn it a million times. I wear it with jeans, slacks, and my silk and chiffon skirts. I am so cool in this jacket.

What's in your underwear drawer?

Thong underwear and camisoles in every one of my colors, plus nude; Hollywood Fashion Tape; my childhood Troll doll Vilhelmina. I have a separate "naughty" drawer that has all the items I put on and take off fairly quickly.

Fashion rules you live by?

I like to stay current with hair and makeup. It keeps me youthful looking without giving the impression I'm trying to be young. I alter my clothing to fit properly. Almost everything I buy needs a tweak. I always check my look with a full-length mirror and use a hand mirror for the back because I don't have a three-way. I'm not kidding.

Rules you break?

I buy T-shirts in not-quite-my-colors. They don't break the bank and the color police are usually on the other side of town when I'm wearing them.

Do you have advice you'd like to pass on?

Search out and buy the best foundations possible for every style of garment you own. Preparedness is bliss. Be true to your own style interpretation, no matter what the masses are doing or saying.

BEAUTY SOAK You've earned a break. Time for a beauty soak, a chance to kick back and have some downtime while immersing yourself in beauty. Go for a walk in a neighborhood park or conservation land and pay attention to the plants, flowers, and trees around you. Observe the beauty in nature, its color combinations and the textures you see — from shiny leaves to fuzzy ones, from solidly colored ones to variegated ones. If there are things you can pick, bring home a bouquet from nature and put it in a pretty vase.

When you've had a nourishing break, come back and we'll begin your resonance book.

✦ ✦ ✦

Chapter 4

RESONANCE

✳

Camp is a structured timeout for yourself. Here you can listen to and look at yourself with a fresh perspective—maybe for the first time in a long time. "Try 'ever,'" you mutter. I heard that! You've been the mother, the best friend, the security blanket. Now you're putting the spotlight on you. If you've been ignoring your needs or desires for a while, then you may have a lot to discover about yourself. You could be as fascinating to yourself as a new best friend.

A resonance book will help you become reacquainted with the real you. It is a collection of anything that moves you right now. It can include words, phrases, and images. You're going to eavesdrop on yourself and find out what really excites and interests you. By collecting these clues and organizing them in one place, you will find it easier to recognize the full picture of who you are right now. It's a powerful tool for honoring yourself and finding your style.

I came up with this idea when I felt really lost and confused. I needed to find a way back to myself, and this really worked. It can work for you, too.

Sometimes life knocks us to our knees and provides an arbitrary halt to normal activities—not the same as this halt you're taking for Beauty Camp, but more like a mud slide that comes off a hill and covers the path in front of you. The natural rhythm of your life temporarily ceases to exist. The event could be divorce, the death of a loved one, or a move to a new community.

I experienced one of those life-halting events when I was diagnosed with breast cancer. My treatment included chemotherapy, surgery, and radiation. As the months went on, I made a point of crossing out every day on my wall calendar as I worked my way to September 1, the day when my treatments would end. I expected that the day after that last black X on my calendar, I'd slide right back into my old life. I'd be doing the exact same things I was doing before I heard those words, "It's cancer."

It didn't happen that way. I was tired. Bone tired. Nothing was comfortable. I felt a letdown. During my treatment I had lots of appointments and made new close friends in the health and healing fields. When those appointments receded, I felt barren. Nothing felt normal. Who was I? Whose life was I living anyway?

One day when I was in my car, I was listening to NPR's radio interview program, *Fresh Air with Terry Gross*. Madonna was on; she was coming out with a new record. She told Terry Gross about her behind-the-scenes collaborations with creative people that she so enjoyed. It was interesting thinking about Madonna working with choreographers, dancers, and lighting technicians. I could appreciate the juicy interactions they must have had. "Collaborations with creative people." Those words hung in the air. I'd been pretty much a loner in my work life, and collaborations with creative people sounded right to me, something I wanted more of in my life. I wrote those four words down on a piece of scrap paper. I wanted to remember them.

One day some friends in the fashion business came over, and we were talking about style. One of them offered, "Brenda, your look is changing. I think you're moving toward a confident, easy, cosmopolitan style." Confident, easy, cosmopolitan. I liked that description! It represented a different way of approaching style for me—dressing in a way that related less to the way people dressed in my own community and more to the world at large, a world I wanted a chance to explore. I wrote the words *confident, easy, cosmopolitan* on a napkin.

The holidays were approaching. I found a card that I just had to take home with me. It was a cartoonlike illustration of a woman riding a red Schwinn bicycle with a basket attached in front that held a small, whimsically decorated Christmas tree. Her beautiful long, brown, wavy hair (it reminded me of the hair I had before chemo took mine away) was blowing behind her as she faced into the wind. She was wearing a long red-and-purple-striped scarf with fringes, pointy-toed spiky heels, and little white fur muffs on her wrists. She had lipstick and eye makeup on (maybe even false eyelashes), and was sitting tall on the bike, looking ahead with a smile on her face.

This image spoke volumes to me. She was a vision of joy and happiness, a lover of fashion and the outdoors. She looked like she was fit, healthy, and loving life. I wanted all of that. I knew that I would never ride a bike in spiked heels. It was a cartoon, after all. But I could see myself breezing down the road of life, feeling fashionable, fit, attractive, and ready for anything—maybe not in a week, but in my near future.

I needed a place to collect these things that spoke to me—this image, and the quotes and ideas that resonated for me. I might have used a journal or a scrapbook, but I decided on a presentation book I already had in my office. It was a 5-by-7-inch bound notebook with about twenty-five plastic-covered pocket pages for slipping in pictures or messages. I put a label on its spine—Resonance Book. Now that I had a place to put these things that were coming to me, I made it a game. I paid attention to anything that I saw or overheard that in my heart I could say yes to. By naming what I loved, what I wanted more of, I was identifying the things that were meaningful to me. Whenever I felt lost, alone, or confused, I'd look at those pages and feel uplifted. I was painting my future.

I was still fatigued, but now this dreaming time was precious to me. I wouldn't wish the experience of going through treatment for cancer on anyone, but

the place it took me to was priceless. My resonance book had become a real lifesaver and a life shaper.

Engage your intuition and imagination for the next week or two and come up with clues to put in a resonance book of your own. (You can use the presentation book you bought when you were shopping for camp.) Be on the lookout for what resonates with you. If you have any doubt about what I mean, consider this: When someone says something that you totally agree with, you can feel the agreement in your gut. In fact, you may even let out a discernible sigh, a signal to you that what you just heard or saw really resonates with you. If a person remarks, "The only way to spend the holidays in December is to go to Mexico" you may know in your gut that is so true for you, even though you haven't done that before. More than anything, you'd like to be in Mexico next December. You can feel the air, smell the ocean, see the drops of moisture on the margarita glasses, taste the salt on the rim. The idea of Mexico in December resonates with you. You're there.

Be bold! Be surprised! Don't brush away a thought that comes into your head. If you get a flash of a red flamingo dress and it doesn't go away, put that in your resonance book. If you start craving cashmere, and in fact you don't want anything else next to your skin but that, put "covered in cashmere" in your book. If a movie star comes to mind, someone from the '40s let's say, and her style resonates with you, find a picture of her for your resonance book. You might visit a card store and look for images that speak to you. Keep your senses awake and alert. This is all about creating a snapshot of you at this moment in time and what you love and want more of in your life. Name your book something else if *resonance book* doesn't, well, resonate with you. Get something to contain your clues. It doesn't have to be precious. It just has to be easy and accessible; you never know when a clue will come to you. They're a gift when they show up, so don't ignore them. Capture them efficiently and put them in a safe spot.

Every time you are tempted to jump back into a rut, you can browse through your resonance book and get recharged and recommitted to honoring the diva within. Dare to reach for the quality of life you've been dreaming of but weren't sure you'd achieve in your lifetime.

Give yourself a big hand for all the great work you're doing. You deserve it! And if you feel like getting out of your jammies and going on a field trip, I invite you to try this exercise: Walk into a store you've never been in before and tell the salesperson you're just looking. Visit every rack and display, from handbags to cocktail dresses. Slowly check out the shoes, jewelry, purses, jackets, blouses, and pants. Owners of a boutique will have items that coordinate with each other. You may realize that you are exactly the right customer for this shop, or you may find nothing that interests you. Either way, you'll begin to learn which stores attract you most.

BEAUTY SOAK Go through your house, gather a few of your very favorite objects, and put them all together in a basket. I want you to remove them from where they usually reside so you can see them with fresh eyes. Sit down in a comfy chair and pull them out one by one. If they have sentimental value, enjoy a long reverie about how you came across them. Give yourself time to daydream about these beautiful things and the quality they add to your life. Sometimes we surround ourselves with beauty but don't take the time to appreciate it. This is your time.

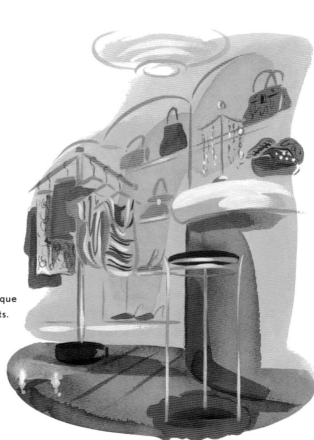

• Visit a new boutique and enjoy the sights.

[Chapter 5]

✦ ✦ ✦

COLOR
YOUR WORLD

❋

Color can turn your world from dowdy to diva faster than anything else. I'll bet there are half a dozen colors that you never dreamed of wearing. You may have heard that redheads can't wear red or that gray-haired women should stay away from gray. There may be colors you automatically avoid because they aren't "your" colors. What if that isn't really true? After working through this chapter, you may be surprised to discover that some of these off-limits colors have become your favorites.

First we'll create a color palette that works because it reflects your own skin, hair, and eye color. For instance, if you have honey-blond hair, a camel coat may look great. If your skin is dark, a rich brown silk scarf may be supreme!

Next we'll look at colors through the eyes of Diva Advisor Randi Merzon, who understands the healing quality of colors. You could start expressing a part of yourself that has lain dormant just by choosing to wear a specific color. For instance, red can awaken you to feelings of passion and power, pink can make you feel loving, and emerald green can put you in touch with your prosperity just by wearing it. Wouldn't it be great to use color like power-juice drinks, as instant pick-me-ups? You can!

In chapters to come, we'll talk about how to bring color into your life—in makeup, clothes, and accessories—to strategically bring out the diva in you. For now, we'll focus on determining which colors are right for you. You won't believe how much easier it is to get dressed when you know the colors in your closet that truly make you shine—even if you're having a rotten, no-good day. (Even divas get the blues!) Ready? Let's go!

If you think you already know what those colors are, don't skip ahead. You may have more to learn. On the other hand, if you feel clueless, that's fine, you won't feel that way for long. By the end of the week, you'll have a personal color palette—a group of colors that make you look and feel great.

First, let's look at how you've been choosing color. This may be one of your biggest ruts. Have you been buying the same color over and over again without really seeing or appreciating any new ones? Or have you been buying every color under the rainbow without paying attention to its effect? Maybe you have lots of color in your wardrobe but things don't really go together. Every fashion season, new colors come into vogue. It can be very confusing trying to figure out which ones you should wear. Let's face it, just because a color is in, it doesn't mean you should be in it.

Personal Coloring

✦ ✦ ✦

I want you to meet a couple of everyday divas. Randi is a robust redhead. She's tall, voluptuous, and forty-seven years old. She has green eyes and her long hair is usually in ringlets. When she wears a copper-colored shawl with an olive green paisley pattern in it, I can't help but stare at her. She's gorgeous!

Debra is fifty-five years old and has silver-gray hair. She's had it since she was in her twenties. Her eyes are dark brown. She is lean and small boned, and her hair is the focal point of her appearance. When she wears white, black, or shades of gray, along with silver jewelry and diamonds, she positively glows.

Randi and Debra have learned how to wear colors that mimic their personal coloring. No matter what colors are fashionable, they'll only spend money on tones that look great on them. If the newest colors don't flatter them, they are content to postpone their shopping until the next season.

Randi and Debra both live in San Francisco, about five miles from each other. Just imagine what would happen if they woke up in each other's bedrooms and got dressed in each other's clothes. They'd look out of step, out of sorts, and completely uncomfortable.

It's worth taking the time to find the colors that make you come alive. If you want professional guidance, you might want to go to your computer right now, type in www.aici.org and find a color consultant near you who can help you understand what colors look best on you. Many members of AICI (Association of Image Consultants International) specialize in color. Even if you see a color consultant and get a color swatch book of forty or so colors, you will still want to make the process of choosing colors simpler and more personal. I'll show you how—with or without a formal color consultation.

Easy Compliments

+ ✦ +

I'm amazed how often it happens. I'll meet a client for the first time, and she'll have an incredible eye color. I'll automatically assume she's taken advantage of this fabulous asset and devoted a third of her closet space to clothes in this color, including shades that are slightly lighter or darker than her eye color. I'll say, "I bet you have clothes in the same color as your eyes, right?" When she looks at me blankly, I know the first thing I'm going to do is dazzle her with this fabulous trick—repeating her eye color in clothing. It's always a wow. The same holds true for hair color, whether it's black, brown, auburn, golden blond, strawberry blond, silver, gray, or white, or has added highlights. When those colors are repeated in clothing pieces the wearer appears sophisticated and confident.

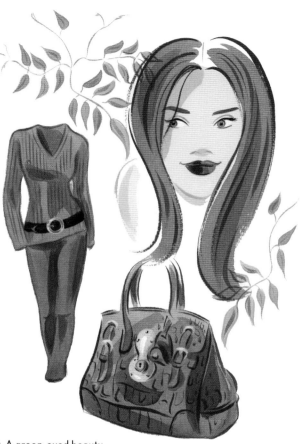

● A green-eyed beauty
wears her signature color.

Women don't often wear colors that mimic their skin tone, but when they do, it's really effective. If your skin tone is dark, wearing a honey-brown dress can feel delicious and free, almost as if you're not wearing anything at all. A fair-skinned person can feel dreamy and yummy in a nude-blush, barely pink, or barely there shade of peach. Watch any red-carpet awards show, and you'll see someone using the color of her skin to a stunning effect. For one thing, wearing your skin tone is a little like going naked. It's so *personal*. Because it copies your skin, it's sexy, seductive, and intimate — especially in soft, fluid fabrics. It can also make one appear vulnerable and soft, which may be great for the woman who is famous for slicing and dicing competitors at the boardroom table, but wants some intimacy with her honey at the dinner table.

Contrast

+ ✦ +

We usually wear outfits that combine two or three colors. Whether you look best in colors that contrast sharply or blend with one another depends on the level of contrast between your skin, hair, and eyes. Is it a high level of contrast, like Snow White's ebony hair, brown eyes, and ivory skin? If that's the case, you can repeat that high level of contrast in your clothing, combining light and dark colors together like black and white, or lemon yellow and deep purple.

Kim, a client of mine, has blond hair with highlights that are even lighter. She has faintly gray-blue eyes. Her level of contrast is very low. She is most comfortable wearing ivory and camel together or pale blue and light taupe.

• **The leather jacket repeats beautiful skin tone color.**

Let me show you how I've used my own coloring and level of contrast to determine my personal colors. My natural hair color is a smoky, dusty brown. I choose to color it to a chestnut brown with caramel highlights. I'm fair skinned and have dark brown eyes. My level of contrast is high. I can wear both light and dark colors and look great. If I stuck with my smoky brown hair color, that level of contrast would not be nearly as high. Colors I love wearing? Black and white, caramel, ivory, and chocolate brown. Those are the beginnings of my personal color palette. They are not the only colors I wear, but they certainly are part of my signature.

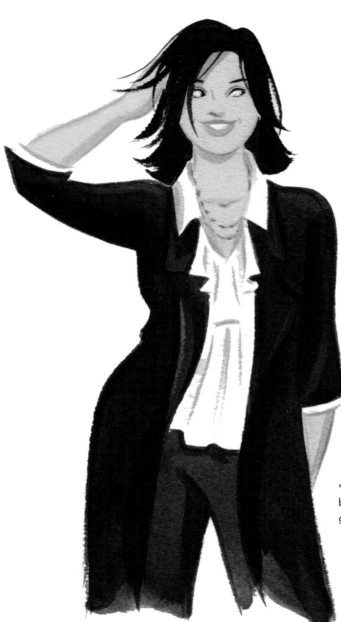

Name Your Colors

✦ ✦ ✦

Take a look in the mirror and write down the colors you see and the level of contrast. If this is hard for you to see or to articulate, ask a good friend, your hairdresser, an interior designer, or a nearby relative to help. When you get the answers, write them below:

Hair:
....

Skin:
....

Eyes:
....

Level of contrast (high, medium, low):
....

Now go to your closet and see if you have colors that echo the colors and contrast level you listed.

• Women with high contrast between their skin and hair look great in high-contrast colors.

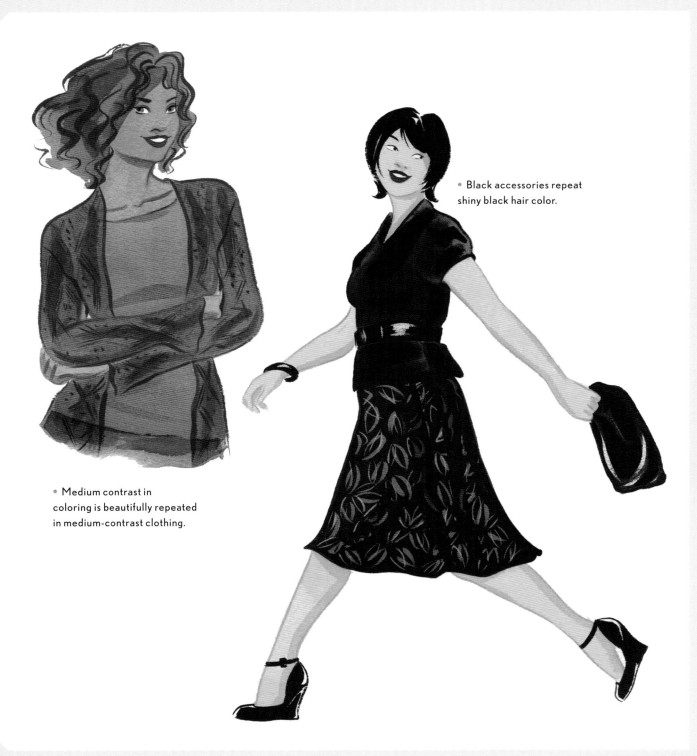

• Black accessories repeat
shiny black hair color.

• Medium contrast in
coloring is beautifully repeated
in medium-contrast clothing.

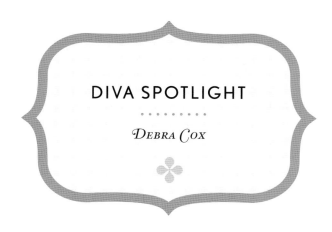

DIVA SPOTLIGHT

Debra Cox

I live in San Francisco. For years I was a very successful entrepreneur, but my life changed dramatically with the death of my husband. It's been two and a half years now, and I'm trying to find my place again. My two daughters both got married this year, four months apart.

What colors do you wear to flatter your natural coloring?
Because I have silver hair, I wear black, white, and charcoal gray.

How do you flatter your assets?
I'm tall and thin and athletic. I like to show off my shoulders, which I do in boatneck tops, off-the-shoulder sweaters, and one-shoulder tops or dresses.

Name a key diva piece.
A great fitting pair of jeans.

What are your must-have accessories?
My Cartier watch, diamond stud earrings, and my most incredible engagement ring, which I now wear on my right hand.

An old favorite that you still wear?
My Loro Piana black cashmere cape.

Name something you splurged on and never looked back.
A Jil Sander coat. The pockets, collar, everything is perfect about it. It's an all-weather coat, perfect for travel, rain repellent, and chic. Oh, and a pair of Manolo Blahnik heels. When I spend a lot on a pair of shoes, it makes my heart pound. But I have no regrets. I have a long narrow foot (size 10N). If the shoe fits and it's practical and sexy, I'll buy it, always in black.

What's in your underwear drawer?
Lots of thongs and always the T-shirt bra with a little padding.

Fashion rules you live by?
I stay true to my style: sophisticated, simple, understated, quality, comfort. When I go outside of this parameter, it's a financial disaster. It's really great to finally get that. If the stores are showing embellished clothing, I don't buy them. I seek out the perfect black top instead. Some seasons I don't buy very much. That's why I wander into the expensive shoe area. When it's a bad shopping time for clothes, I buy shoes, handbags, and sunglasses.

Rules you break?
Not everything has to be a good buy. I'll spend a little on something I'll wear once or twice. If I spend a lot of money on something, I'll want to wear it a lot.

Do you have advice you'd like to pass on?
Wear sunscreen.

Warm and Cool

+ ✦ +

Another way to find flattering colors is to determine whether you wear cool or warm colors best, or whether you can wear both. Again, you'll be looking at your own coloring to determine this. Let me be clear about my terms: You often hear people say blue and green are cool colors, while red and orange are warm. When I talk about warm and cool colors, I'm applying those labels to all colors. Among all the possible shades of blue, there are warm blues and cool blues. The same goes for green, red, yellow, and so on. Warm colors have golden undertones. Cool colors have blue undertones. Here are some warm and cool examples of colors. In the first line, tomato red has a golden undertone, which makes it warm. Bordeaux red, a wine color, has a blue undertone, which makes it cool.

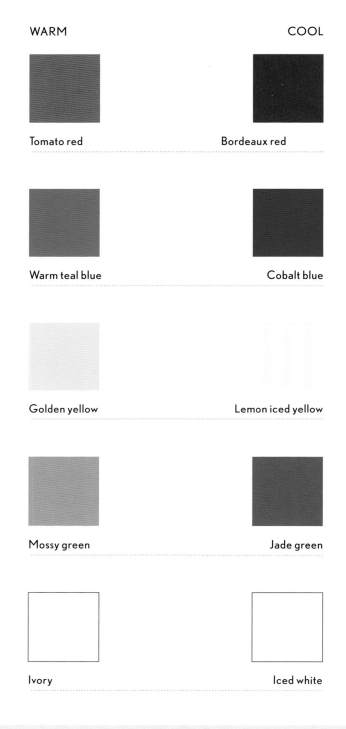

WARM   COOL

Tomato red   Bordeaux red

Warm teal blue   Cobalt blue

Golden yellow   Lemon iced yellow

Mossy green   Jade green

Ivory   Iced white

Here's a helpful and fun exercise. Go to the scarf department at your favorite store and pull scarves off the shelves in both warm and cool tones. Standing in front of a full-length mirror in good light (very important!), hold them up under your chin, one by one. If the light is good, it can be quite easy to see which colors make you look vital, youthful, and exciting, and which colors make you look tired, heavy, gloomy, or sad. It's really quite a dramatic exercise!

You may respond to cool, saturated colors in a scarf — ruby red, royal blue, emerald green, purple. Or you may look better in a scarf with cool, muted colors, such as raspberry red, sea foam green, and French blue. You may want to buy a multicolored scarf to keep as a reference for what collection of colors looked best on you — a color palette, in other words.

Or gather together scarves that belong to neighbors and friends and find yourself a full-length mirror in good light and see what colors make you look healthier and more vital. You can make this a beauty soak expedition. Write down some colors you want to explore and put your notes in your diva journal. Add to it colors that you've gotten compliments on. Sometimes we're the last to figure out what looks good, so listen up. Use those detective skills you learned while putting together your resonance book.

Trolling for Color

✦ ✦ ✦

What I've been giving you so far are guidelines — good ones. Now let's look at another level of color exploration, based on your intuition. Before you buy a single thing, I'd like you to capture the color and style ideas you want to explore. I know we haven't officially started to discuss style, so for now let's keep it simple and fun. I don't want to limit your intuition to only color. Let your eyes feast on and collect whatever you love, and we'll sort everything out later.

What you'll need is a stack of magazines. You'll be tearing out pages that feature colors, patterns, and styles that inspire you. Current fashion magazines will have the latest color palettes and silhouettes that designers are using, but they're not necessary. You can go through back issues of fashion, garden, or home design magazines and get great results. Later you can decide whether you want to organize your tear sheets on a piece of poster board or in a scrapbook.

Before you start tearing through magazines looking for pictures of what you love, take a few minutes to clear your mind. Take a few deep breaths. You know, you hardly ever get to just think about yourself, so don't rush through this. Take time to get in the mood.

Let go of any ideas you have about color or style. For now, I would like you to forget the discussions we just had about high and low contrast, and warm and cool colors. Clear your mind of everything that's in your closet, too, even your most recent purchases. In this exercise, don't second-guess the pictures you pull. Don't ask yourself, "Is that a color I could wear?"

"Could I wear that style of pant?" "Would that blouse look good on me?" Let your heart take the lead. Let go of all the rules you've ever heard—"blonds look good in black; dark colors make you look thinner; don't wear white after Labor Day; buy taupe because it goes with everything." Cleanse your visual palette. Cleanse your emotional palette as well. Ready?

Go through the magazines one by one and tear out pictures of things you love. Don't edit them. Just pay attention to what you love. It could be color combinations, specific jacket styles, the way jewelry is combined, anything. You're a kid in a candy store. This is where the ideas start. You might even come across some word messages, some advertising jingles or headlines that resonate for you. Grab those too!

With your stack of pulled pictures, get out a pair of scissors and cut out what thrills you about each and every page. Now group the pictures by color. Do you have lots of pictures of one color, or a family of colors? Did you end up pulling pictures of colors that repeat your skin, hair, and eye colors? Any surprises? Notice if there seems to be a color that you feel especially hungry for. What is it? Are you surprised? Remember, we're not doing anything yet, just collecting ideas and inspiration. Move your tear sheets around on a table or on the floor and just observe what you see. Then gather them together and store them in a safe place, such as your binder or a folder.

I'm going to end this section with a list of colors and the messages or qualities that are associated with them as given to us by Diva Advisor Randi Merzon—yes, the same Randi with the gorgeous red hair (page 50)!

THE HEALING PROPERTIES OF COLOR

BY RANDI MERZON

Randi Merzon is an intuitive counselor who utilizes color as a healing force for change.

You can use color to lift your mood or inspire you. Lost your grounding? Feeling unsettled? Wear something in rust, honey, amber, or forest green. Don't have the time for meditation today? Try a color meditation. Simply attune yourself to the healing qualities of the colors and fabrics in your clothes. Allow each color's vibration to remind you all day long of the power it holds. Remember how it feels when you buy that first bunch of yellow daffodils after a dreary winter? Wear daffodil yellow and allow your energy to become attuned to that color; you're likely to feel an extra spring in your step.

Surround yourself with colors you love. Begin to practice your color intuition: When you wake up in the morning, what are the colors that speak to you first? Ask yourself, "How do I want to feel today?" Then choose the color that will reinforce that feeling (see the list of colors and their qualities on the following page).

Colors and Their Attributes

✦ ✦ ✦

•• Blue ••

Sky blue — sensitivity, spirituality, expansiveness

Royal blue — physical strength

Cobalt blue — calm

Aqua — calm

Turquoise — humor, playfulness

Aquamarine — peacefulness

•• Green ••

Emerald green — prosperity

Forest green — prosperity and abundance

Apple green — new growth, new beginnings

•• Yellow ••

Lemon yellow — mental clarity

Buttercream yellow — harmony, self-love, abstract intuition

•• Orange ••

Citrus orange — creative expression

Burnt orange/rust — body healing, vitality

Terra-cotta — rootedness

Peach — healing

•• Red ••

Fire-engine red — passion, courage, vitality

Brick red — rootedness, calm

•• Pink ••

Fuchsia — love and caring, creative inspiration

Pink — love, affinity, compassion

•• Purple ••

Lavender — spirituality, self-acceptance

Purple — spiritual inquiry and study

•• Metallic ••

Copper — spiritual uplift

Silver — personal power

Gold — harmony, wisdom

Pearly white or opalescent — integrated sense of spirituality

A special note about metallics such as gold, silver, bronze, and copper. Metallics make you feel more in harmony with the universe at large. They also make you feel like a million bucks. Metallics remind you not to be afraid to come out and shine and be who you are.

You're on a roll. You're moving past your ruts, toward the things that resonate with you. You're seeing color in a new exciting way. Let's keep your intuition and creativity engaged and move into the next chapter, where we'll start defining your diva style.

BEAUTY SOAK Go on a color expedition around your house and come back with samples of colors you love. There may be color clues three feet away from you. Artists and designers were paid well to design the color palettes that exist in your sheets, shower curtains, dishes, and rugs, as well as the gift-wrap paper and greeting cards you've stashed away. If you are in love with the rug on your floor, look closely at the colors. Would they work on you? Look at the things you naturally collect, such as earthenware or blue glass. Look at the colors you've painted your walls. Often the colors of things we surround ourselves with in our homes are the same ones we would love wearing. Snip samples of these colors wherever you can and keep them in your binder or in a folder. Or, in the case of a rug, see if you can collect samples of the colors from other sources, such as paint samples, colored paper, or magazines, and put them together in a color palette.

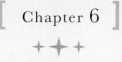

[Chapter 6]

✦ ✦ ✦

DEFINING
YOUR
DIVA STYLE

✳

You've got style. How do I know?
Because inside of everyone is her style
DNA. Yours is made up of the things
you love and what you want others to
know about you. When you're dressed
in clothes and accessories that match
your style DNA, you're a dynamo.
You feel confident, complete, satiated.
It's heaven; let's get you there.

Tic-Tac-Toe Style Games

✦ ✦ ✦

In order to help you identify your style, I'm going to have you do some style testing. It shouldn't take too much time and it's as simple as tic-tac-toe. You may have read articles or books about style suggesting you are one of five basic types: conservative, dramatic, sexy, sporty, or creative. I don't subscribe to this method of defining women's style because it's so narrow and uninspiring. Your unique style is far more fascinating. These exercises will help you see yourself much more clearly. Get a few sheets of paper and a pencil. Ready?

•• My Favorite Things ••

Go around your house and pick between five and ten of your very favorite things. It would be best if they were portable so you can gather them and review them as a group. They might include a piece of china, a knickknack, pillow, painting, pretty perfume bottle—you get the picture. Put them on a cleared tabletop. (Or, if you have a favorite room in your house where you love everything about it, go there now with your pencil and paper.) Make a tic-tac-toe grid on your paper covering the whole page. In the center write "My Favorite Things." Now, looking at the items you grouped together, report objectively on the quality of the items as if you were a journalist or a detective. In each of the remaining spaces of the grid—there will be eight of them—write in the adjectives that describe your favorite things. You might use words like *elegant*,

luxurious, fun, cozy, dramatic, grand, regal, whimsical, poetic, and *charming*. You can put in more than one word per box if you need to. Even though you're looking at several different objects, they may share the same characteristics. When you feel you've captured the essence of these objects, put this page aside and get ready to do another one.

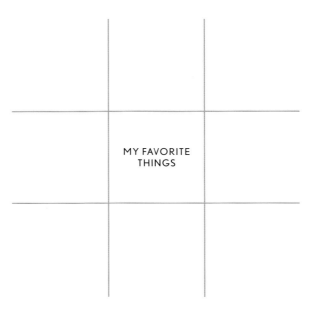

MY FAVORITE
THINGS

•• What I Love ••

Go to your closet or dressing area. Look through your clothes and accessories and pick out ten items that you just love. They might be a strand of pearls, pair of earrings, skirt, jacket, shoe, blouse, coat—anything that you adore. Lay them all out on your couch and coffee table or spread them across your cleared dining room table. If they stay in the closet, they'll just look like clothes. Look at them with your detective eyes. What is it you love about these items? Using the

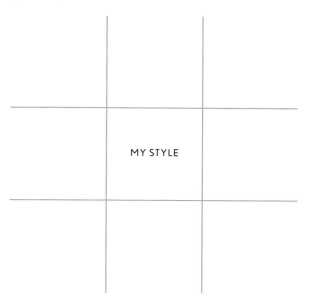

	WHAT I LOVE	

you liked about it, throw it away. Write "My Style" in the center of a fresh tic-tac-toe grid. Now, acting like a detective again, look at the pictures and describe the qualities you see.

	MY STYLE	

tic-tac-toe grid, write "What I Love" in the center of it and in the remaining eight boxes, fill in the adjectives. You may use words like *retro, modern, old-fashioned, glamorous, striking, flirty, pretty,* or *bold*, for example. Use phrases if one word won't do, for example, *feminine with a twist, moody and mysterious, earthy opulence.* Your pieces may once again express similar qualities. That's fine. Leave these things out for a few hours. When you bump into them unexpectedly, something might strike you about them that you missed before. Double up words in the boxes if you need to. Set this aside and go to the next activity.

·· My Style ··

Grab the pictures you cut out of magazines. Find a surface where you can spread them out. When you look at them again, be sure you still love them. If you're looking at a page and wondering what it was

Terrific. You're going to evaluate these three grids. Before you do, take a quick walk around the block, dance to some music, sing a song—do something that will clear your mind and release the concentration you've held.

When you've taken a revitalizing break, grab a cup of tea or some coffee and find your favorite spot to sit down and analyze these exercises. This is a creative process. The information on these sheets will lead you to your style DNA. Look at all three pages. Do you see similarities among the answers? Is there some overlap? I would expect there would be. Make a list of the words and phrases you noted. Read it to yourself. Do the words resonate with you? If someone was describing you and used those words, would you feel flattered?

When you read the list, you should be able to say unequivocally, "Yes, that's really me! I love these qualities! If my fashion style reflected these qualities, I'd be happy, happy, happy."

If there are some adjectives that don't resonate with you, delete them from your list. If there are some qualities that give you butterflies, like the word *sophisticated*, all to the good. It means you're ready to do some stretching. I like that!

If you don't see any connections, try doing the exercises again with other objects and clothing pieces. You can always get help with this part, too. Invite a friend or a loved one to be a detective and tell you what he or she sees about your objects, your clothes, or your tear outs. It might be easier to see them through someone else's eyes.

DIVA SENSE

"I'd like my wardrobe to be like my place. My home is subtle. You might miss the care that went in to choosing the things I display, but as you look at them more closely, you really appreciate them. I'd like my clothes to be appreciated the same way. I'd like you to look at how I've put things together and say to yourself, 'Oh, that's an interesting person.' I don't want someone to look at me and say 'Oh, she's wearing Armani.'
Marilyn

Select-o-Style
✦ ✦ ✦

I heard the actor Alan Alda being interviewed about his role as a powerful senator on the TV show *The West Wing*. "How did you do it?" the interviewer asked. Alda replied, "I shook hands with the part of me that's powerful and at ease about it." I'm convinced we have many parts of ourselves. Up until now, you may have expressed a fraction of yourself, and now you're ready to explore more. Did you come across some qualities that surprised you in the exercises? I hope so. If not, you have another chance. Your style, at this stage of your life, should include parts of yourself that you're ready to shake hands with.

More Words about Style
✦ ✦ ✦

Read through this list of more than fifty words and circle any that aren't on your other lists, but are calling out to you. Add them to your list of style words.

Review your entire list of words. See if anything needs to be dropped. The reason you'd drop something is because you've spent enough time on a quality and you're ready to move on to something you haven't explored as much. Maybe you've chosen *classic* as a signature style for years. Even though you still have a lot of that in you, you also have *lusciousness, playfulness,* and *spirituality,* which you want to express. Move *classic* aside for a bit while you explore these other qualities.

I want you to feel really excited about your words. Review your resonance book. You may have noted some words or phrases that fit your style DNA exactly.

Take some of your key words and look them up in the dictionary. For instance, if *sassy* is on your list, the dictionary may define it as "lively and spirited." Maybe *lively* and *spirited* are closer to what you meant. Finding just the right words to describe your style is worth some time with a dictionary. Go for exactly what you want.

fearless	*soft*	*exciting*	*sassy*
exuberant	*juicy*	*creative*	*bubbly*
radiant	*healthy*	*interesting*	*strong*
adorable	*sporty*	*feminine*	*surprising*
luscious	*available*	*arty*	*good-humored*
powerful	*warm*	*seductive*	*exotic*
vivacious	*innovative*	*original*	*well traveled*
sexy	*magnetic*	*sensual*	*energetic*
rich	*eye-candy*	*poised*	*opulent*
classy	*ravishing*	*gracious*	*luxurious*
fun-loving	*stunning*	*ladylike*	*sparkly*
welcoming	*sultry*	*succulent*	*captivating*
vibrant	*attractive*	*sweet*	*peaceful*
alive	*pretty*	*organic*	*spiritual*

Your style DNA is specific to you. If you've gathered a dozen or so words, see if you can distill them down to six words. If you can't, that's fine. Work with the list you've made but review it and see if you feel the same about it tomorrow, next week, and two weeks from now. This is a process. Keep a copy of the list in your purse. Put another copy on your closet door. These words are precious. They could make you shriek in delight or weep at being seen so clearly. Let your style words rest in your heart. Take time to own them.

Your Beauty Box

Congratulations! You've identified your style! Take time to celebrate. Take a break from your exercises and build your own personal beauty reminder box. It will sustain you next week when you're in your closet moving out your unwanted clothes. I want you to collect things of beauty that delight you. Make them everyday kinds of things, not priceless knickknacks. These are most likely small enough to fit into a shoebox, cigar box, or recycled stationery box. When you gaze into your beauty box, you'll feel refreshed and reminded of what stirs you. You might include postcards or greeting cards that are especially beautiful or symbolic to you. You might have ribbons in beautiful colors, small illustrations, empty perfume bottles, and other little treasures that mean something to you. These cherished objects can help you appreciate what's unique about you when you are busy and harried. It's good to have a place to come back to, to appreciate your aesthetic. Soon your clothes will remind you of that as well, but until then, keep this in a visible place so you can look at it often.

Color and Style Together

✦ ✦ ✦

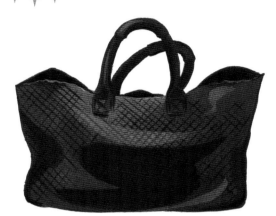

• **A red bag adds excitement to any outfit.**

Color and style make a great team. How you use color in your outfits may be a big component of your style formula. If you're going to be famous for being mysterious, orange or yellow probably won't be the colors you choose. No, you'll want murky navy blues, questionable blacks—any color that is close to, but not exactly, black. Or color could be a way that you express your daring self. French fashion designer Elsa Schiaparelli was famous for wearing shocking pink, her signature color, which was very daring for her time. There was no mistaking the power of Nancy Reagan, who became famous for wearing red while in the White House. The colors you choose to wear play a distinctive role in your signature style. Will you be dramatic in all one color, head to toe? Will you mix two unexpected colors to demonstrate your creativ-

ity? Will you want to look soft and feminine, wearing neutral shades of taupe, but than add a surprise in a bright pink handbag? Head-to-toe yellow may be over the top, but a yellow leather jacket may be a key piece that supports your playfulness.

My copper-haired friend Marj puts color and style together in a pair of peach suede pants that really suits her. Peach works beautifully with her coloring and the soft suede relates to her ultrafeminine style. Then she adds a pair of ankle-strap peach satin heels, and she's even more feminine and sexy! How many people will have peach suede pants in their closet? It's definitely a key diva piece of hers.

Lynn, a colleague, maximizes the drama of color with a one-two color punch. She wears a green scoop-neck T-shirt under a black off-the-shoulder T-shirt. She adds a double strand of beads in jet black, jade green, and rusty red (carnelian). Then she finishes off the outfit with a black asymmetrical skirt that is shorter in the front, and a pair of black boots. By repeating the black and green in both her necklace and her T-shirts, she creates a magnetic attraction between the two colors. It's hard to take your eyes off this stunning combination.

Before we start putting clothes together that support your style, let's do another tic-tac-toe exercise. In the center of the grid write "My Colors." In the eight empty boxes, write the colors you adore and would love to wear. They could be colors from the personal palette you worked on in the last chapter plus some new ones. For inspiration, look around your house, at the objects you collected to do your style exercises, or even at your favorite things in your closet. You can also go back through the stack of pages you've ripped out of magazines and see if there are any colors there that you'd like to consider. Remember metallic colors, too. If you run out of space going around the grid, double up. When you look at your tic-tac-toe grid, you should see all the colors you'd like to consider using in your wardrobe and in your outfits. Mentally overlay the colors with your style words and see how color can bring out your words. If *fun* and *lively* were in your list of style words and orange and red appear in your color tic-tac-toe, you're definitely on the right track! This isn't an exercise in practicality. You're still in the discovery phase. You may not wear blue-green very well next to your face, but in a handbag it might be perfect. So don't rule anything out. Just love these colors.

MY COLORS

When you work within a palette of color, putting outfits together and shopping for key diva pieces are a breeze. Gone are the days of buying the same top in every color. You don't need to. You only need to buy things in the palette you're working with.

Here are a few ready-made palettes that I've created. You might want to lean on one that seems closest to the direction you're moving in while you continue to explore color. If you look back at your tear sheets or at the personal color palette you started based on your coloring, you may find that one of these palettes is a good jumping-off point from which to define and refine the colors you like. Remember, color and style put together strategically will really set you apart. You will become excited about choosing color rather than settling or making do with something that's boring and dowdy.

·· Serene and Refined ··

COLORS:

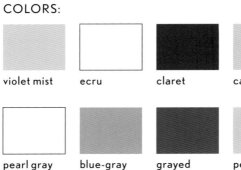

violet mist   ecru   claret   camel

 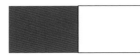 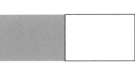 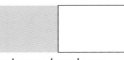

pearl gray   blue-gray   grayed green   pearl green

COLOR COMBOS:

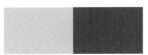

claret / violet mist

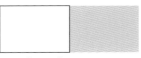

blue-gray / pearl gray

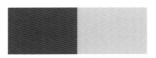

grayed green / ecru

pearl green / pearl gray

camel / grayed green

ecru / camel

grayed green / pearl green

blue-gray / camel

·· Creative and Rich ··

COLORS:

apple green   egg shell   brick red   moss

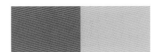 

wine   curry   avocado   teal

COLOR COMBOS:

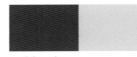

teal / apple green

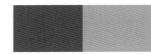

brick red / curry

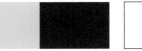

avocado / moss

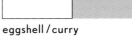

wine / curry

apple green / wine

eggshell / curry

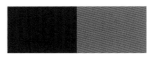

teal / eggshell

wine / brick red

•• Warm and Spicy ••

•• Cool and Natural ••

COLORS:

| vanilla | nutmeg | chile red | raspberry |

| lentil | ginger | spruce | turmeric |

COLORS:

| white | cornflower blue | cool gray | misty green |

| lavender | putty | soft blue | slate blue |

COLOR COMBOS:

raspberry / turmeric

lentil / spruce

ginger / spruce

turmeric / vanilla

lentil / vanilla

raspberry / chile red

raspberry / nutmeg

ginger / nutmeg

COLOR COMBOS:

cool gray / soft blue

lavender / slate blue

putty / white

cornflower blue / putty

misty green / putty

cool gray / cornflower blue

white / soft blue

slate blue / cool gray

•• Light and Spirited ••

COLORS:

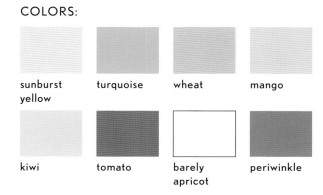

sunburst yellow   turquoise   wheat   mango

kiwi   tomato   barely apricot   periwinkle

COLOR COMBOS:

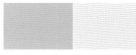 turquoise / sunburst yellow

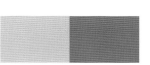 wheat / tomato

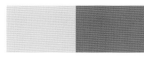 mango / tomato

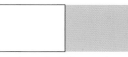 barely apricot / turquoise

 kiwi / tomato

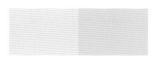 sunburst yellow / mango

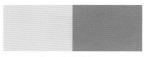 mango / periwinkle

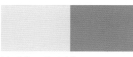 kiwi / periwinkle

•• Royal Opulence ••

COLORS:

purple   bright red   golden yellow   black

emerald   white   deep purple   gold

COLOR COMBOS:

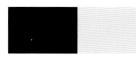 black / golden yellow

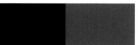 black / bright red

 bright red / deep purple

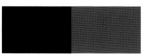 black / purple

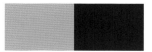 gold / deep purple

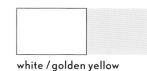 emerald / deep purple

 white / golden yellow

golden yellow / bright red

•• Feminine and Classic ••

COLORS:

 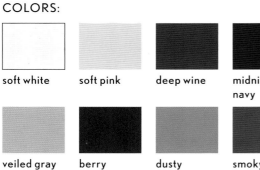 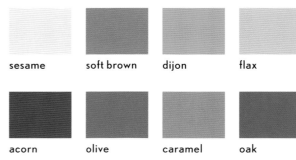

soft white   soft pink   deep wine   midnight navy

veiled gray   berry   dusty amethyst   smoky forest green

COLOR COMBOS:

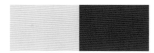 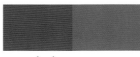

soft pink / deep wine   smoky forest green / soft white

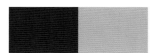 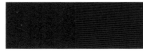

midnight navy / veiled gray   berry / midnight navy

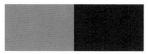 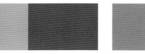

dusty amethyst / berry   soft white / deep wine

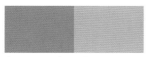 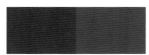

dusty amethyst / veiled gray   deep wine / smoky forest green

•• Organic and Botanical ••

COLORS:

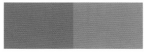 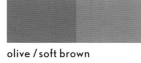

sesame   soft brown   dijon   flax

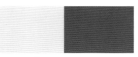

acorn   olive   caramel   oak

COLOR COMBOS:

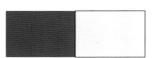 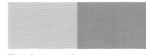

acorn / oak   olive / soft brown

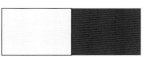 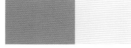

flax / caramel   sesame / acorn

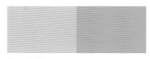 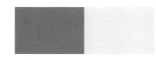

dijon / acorn   soft brown / sesame

olive / sesame   flax / dijon

There's one more tic-tac-toe exercise to do: This one is about fabric and texture. You may have noticed when gathering objects and pictures that you are really attracted to certain patterns, textures, finishes, images, or details. Create a grid to explore what you love in this area. Write "Patterns, Textures, Finishes, Images, Details" in the center box. You may be drawn to the fabric itself or the treatment on the fabric like quilting, embroidery, or appliqué. Consider things like satin, lace, sequins, jacquard, brocade, linen, silk, rubber, crinkled linen, crushed velvet, denim, plaids, paisleys, polka dots, stripes, and floral prints. Maybe you have a thing for butterflies or Chinese temples. If you do have an image or symbol that you really love, be sure to add it to your grid. If you fill in the eight boxes and have more to add, keep going around your grid until you capture all the things you love in fabrics.

It's time to round up your good ideas and organize them in a binder. You should have a list of style words and images to go with them; a group of colors that you'd like to work with and images that support those; and you should have a list of patterns, textures, finishes, and details that you really love, and images that reflect them. This wealth of information about the things you love will be your guide as you put together outfits for your three dates. Keep referring to it. This is your style DNA. It doesn't match anyone else's.

To organize your information visually, go through your color and style sample pictures, trim them up, and paste them onto black construction paper. Then slide them into sheet protectors that will go into your three-ring binder. You might organize a page just for color and a page just for patterns, textures, finishes, images, and details. You will be amazed how soothing, comforting, and enjoyable it is to just look at these pages. Or, if you like making collages on poster board, you might prefer to mount your pictures rather than put them in a binder. Do what works for you.

	PATTERNS TEXTURES FINISHES IMAGES DETAILS	

Diva Sense

"I have learned that if something doesn't feel good on my skin, I won't wear it. I don't want to wear anything that's hard or scratchy. I may pay more for something that feels luxurious, but I've found it saves me money in the end. It's cheaper to own a few things that I love wearing than to buy inexpensive stuff that doesn't meet my 'feel' standards and then never gets worn."

Mary

You've been focusing on your style and the things you love. Now ask yourself this question: "If I could have more of what I love, what would it be?" Imagine a boutique that was filled with only the clothes and accessories that delight you. What would line the shelves or hang on the racks? Let your imagination go. I think you know what would be there. Consider pants, skirts, dresses, coats, shoes, and accessories. Each piece should express your style and give you pure enjoyment. Start your list on a sheet of paper and put it in your binder when you're done.

In Brenda's Boutique, here are some of the things that are on the shelves and on the racks:

+ Important necklaces that are beautiful, feminine, and glamorous

+ Really pretty earrings

+ Lovely, feminine tops that are lacy and thin but not see-through, in fabrics that feel good against my body

+ Playful jackets in luxury fabrics

+ An array of beautiful shawls and fun scarves that I can wear with many things

+ Sexy pants—close fitting to the butt and legs

+ All sorts of clothing in happy colors like yellow, turquoise, and orange, and in luscious colors like creamy vanilla, cinnamon, and soft gold

+ Swishy, feminine skirts

+ Sexy bare shoes that look good with fresh pedicures

This list lets me assess what I have already and it allows me to see where I need to grow my wardrobe so it matches what I really love. Review your list. What does it tell you? Write down your thoughts and comments in your diva journal now.

You've taken the time to figure out your style. You've started thinking about how you'd express it by doing your boutique exercise. And you haven't tried on a single piece of clothing. Good!

Soon, you're going to be spending quite a bit of time in your closet. You're going to be moving things out of there and maybe getting your nose filled with musty, dusty smells. Before we get to that, plan for a day of rest and relaxation—anytime soon is good! Diva Advisor Victoria Katayama has a tried-and-true plan for arranging a spa day right in your home. If it seems too elaborate, she also has suggestions for "spa day lite." Follow her lead for some revitalization.

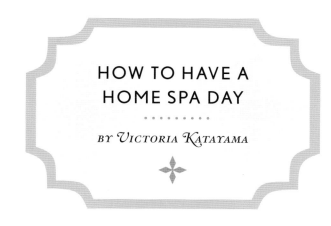

HOW TO HAVE A HOME SPA DAY

·········

BY VICTORIA KATAYAMA

✦

Victoria Katayama is the owner of Relax Simply, a business centered around relaxation and relaxation products.

You don't have to travel to another city, state, or country in order to have a pampering spa experience. You can have one right at home! Here are the steps to take to give yourself a much-needed break from the pace and responsibilities of a busy life and enjoy some rejuvenation. Spa time is fun in numbers. Get some friends together (no more than five) or invite your sisters. Send other family members away for the day. Gather for a wonderful breakfast, complete with French pastries, lattes, and fresh fruit, all served on beautiful china. Surround yourself with lots of fragrant bouquets of flowers.

Arrange to have up to three massage therapists come over to give treatments, including salt scrubs, massage, Lomi-Lomi (an ancient Hawaiian massage), and Watsu (shiatsu massage done in very warm water). Massage tables can be set up outside in the fresh air under a canopy of trees for shade, and the Watsu could be done in your swimming pool if you have one. Proceed through the day receiving wonderful treatments and lounging in between, reading your favorite magazines, talking, or just resting.

For dinner have a local chef prepare a gourmet meal. He or she can use your kitchen to prepare the meal, and then serve you. Linger over the meal for hours, talk, laugh, and share your darkest secrets all night long. Guaranteed, you'll drift off to sleep relaxed and happy.

To set up your spa day you will need to do the following:

1. Set aside a whole day.

2. Book the massage therapists in advance. Find out what treatments they offer — types of massage, scrubs, and wraps. Communicate to the massage therapists clearly what everyone wants in advance so they can bring the necessary items for the treatments.

3. Make sure you have all the supplies you will need, such as extra towels for showering after treatments, rose petals for the massage table, and special products that you want to use or that the therapists have recommended.

4. Ask everyone to bring robes or comfortable clothing and slippers to lounge in.

5. Prepare or buy great healthful food and drinks in advance so you keep your energy level up.

Before you open your spa:

1. Fill a pitcher of water with sliced lemon or lime and make it available during the day.

2. Place rose petals on the massage tables.

3. Place a small bowl of flowers under the face-cradle of the massage table so you can smell and see them while on the table.

4. Set the mood with relaxing music playing, candles, and fresh fragrant flowers.

SPA DAY LITE

Are you interested in a spa day on a smaller scale? A great alternative would be to spend a day of relaxing alone or with a special person in your life. Set aside a whole day and plan a spa getaway at home.

Start with a delicious array of your favorite breakfast foods and beverages, served on beautiful china. Surround yourself with lots of fragrant bouquets of flowers.

After breakfast, take a leisurely walk in a place that brings you joy, such as the woods, a pretty garden, or an ocean beach.

When you return, give yourself a facial steam: Boil water and pour it into a pretty heatproof bowl. Add a few drops of your favorite essential oil (available at health food stores), or some sprigs of lavender, rosemary, or mint, or the zest and juice of a lemon or orange. Bend over the bowl, put a towel over your head, and breathe in the fresh aromas as you revitalize your skin.

Next draw a nice, warm bubble bath and toss in fragrant fresh flower petals, such as rose or gardenia. Surround the tub with candles and have your favorite soothing music playing in the background.

While you're still in the tub, exfoliate your skin with the scrub you prepared (see step 4): To polish your skin, simply lift a leg or arm out of the water, scrub, and put it back.

After your bath, rest quietly in a place that makes you happy, such as the garden or deck.

Later, go out to dinner at your favorite place, prepare a delicious meal yourself, or order food from your favorite take-out restaurant. If eating at home, have fun arranging a beautiful table setting in advance so it feels special when you sit down to eat. Enjoy!

To set this up, this is what you need to do:

1. Set aside a whole day.

2. Make sure you have all the necessary supplies for the treatments (extra towels, special products you want to use, music, etc.).

3. Set up your facial steam area and make it look beautiful.

4. Make your scrub: Mix 1 cup of sea salt with 1 cup of olive oil in a medium-size bowl. Add the zest and juice of an orange or lemon or your favorite essential oil.

5. Set the mood with relaxing music playing, candles, and fresh fragrant flowers.

6. Have robes or comfortable clothing and slippers to lounge in.

7. Have plenty of soft towels.

8. Prepare or buy great, healthful food and drinks in advance.

9. Have a pitcher of water with sliced lemons or limes available during the day.

BEAUTY SOAK Visit an art museum, go to the library and look at art history books, or purchase high-quality art books with paintings by great artists. Go through them looking for what appeals to you most. Do you love the soft colors of some Impressionists? The dark colors of some of the Romantics? The bold colors of the Modernists? Are you delighted by the rich color palette from a Dutch still life of pomegranates, pumpkin, and red and green grapes? Can you focus on what the models are wearing and appreciate details about their clothing? Feast your eyes on art and see if there's a palette that inspires you, or a mood that you can relate to style.

• For absolute luxury, soak in gardenias on your well-deserved spa day.

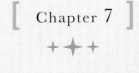

[Chapter 7]

✦ ✦ ✦

FIT FOR A DIVA

Before we head into your closet to find your diva things and ditch your dowdy ones, there's one more piece of the puzzle to address, and that is *fit*—the assets and challenges of your figure. We'll be working with fit next week in your closet and again when you're shopping in Week Three. There are some things you can be thinking about now, however, before you try on clothes and assess your image in front of a full-length mirror.

Before we go near this subject, I need a commitment from you. I want you to be nice. We've had a lot of fun. We've played around with colors and enjoyed some games while discovering your style. You're closer than ever to expressing the diva inside of you. And now we're going to be talking about your body. If you're like most women, you're probably pretty mean when it comes to your body. You complain about it. It's not the one you want. It used to be better (but you complained about it then, too). Now it's changing and you don't know what to do. When you talk about your body, being nice and being curious about what it needs right now probably don't come naturally to you. That's where I come in. Listen to me and follow my lead. I'm going to give you lots of tips on how your body will enjoy being dressed, and how good fit can make you feel wonderful and add to the already great things that are happening for you with color and style.

DIVA SENSE

"My weight has rearranged itself, and somehow my waist has expanded. I used to have a slim waist. And now I have boobs that I never had before. It's really unfair. I've had a hissy fit all year. I walk for half an hour every day. I go to the gym, I get exercise. I don't suddenly have a very sedentary life. I want to adapt to my state of being and stop sulking inside, saying 'It's unfair.' I want to get to 'this is where I am, it's fine, let's go from here.'" *Marilyn*

Adjust

✦ ✦ ✦

Everyone has her own particular shape. No amount of wishing for a different one is going to change the one you have. Complaining about your shape is like complaining about the weather. It's not going to change a thing. You're still going to need a jacket for warmth, a raincoat or umbrella if it's raining, or a hat and sunscreen if you're headed for the beach. You adapt to the conditions. The same holds true for your body. There are certain things you can do to accommodate it.

In the previous chapters you've learned that there's so much more to you and your look than shape. There's color, and there's style. When you apply these to clothes that flatter your own personal shape, there's no stopping you. Women get all squirmy talking about fit. It helps to remember that fit is just one-third of the formula we're going for — color, style, fit, or CSF for short. CSF sounds like a new TV crime show, right? No, it's just a quick way for you to remember what it takes to be looking like the diva you are. When you walk out the door having those three elements lined up, you're as dynamic as the star of any show, only this one is your show! Bad fit brings attention to itself. Good fit brings attention to you. Not enough people have it or demand it, but you will. I'll teach you how.

Some Surprises

✦✦✦

If you've put the pleasure of wearing clothes you love on hold because you don't have the right body size, meet someone who used to think the same way. Mary was somewhere between a size 14 and 18. She had a trainer and a plan to lose weight, but it wasn't dropping off as quickly as she hoped. She had dreams of what she'd wear when she was thin. In the meantime, her strategy was to be invisible. It was hard for her to understand that her figure was an incredible asset, something she should be showing off, not hiding. She was well toned, had great proportion, and a really cute body. She was convinced that she needed to wear black or navy blue all the time because of her "weight." I wish you could have seen her face when I brought a pair of red Capri pants to her dressing room. I'm sure she thought she'd hired a kook; I could see her looking for the nearest exit. "I know it's not what you were expecting, but just try them on for fun," I said. We spent a long time in front of the three-way mirror outside the dressing room area. The pants were so flattering on her. Her cute round butt was adorable in them. The proportions were great.

Mary feared that the red pants would look like a red fire truck coming down the street. Like most of us, in her mind she greatly magnified the body parts she's most self-conscious about. "This would be great to wear on weekends with a white T-shirt and a jean jacket and some flip-flops," I said. I kept talking. I thought the longer I talked and explained what I was seeing, the better the chances were that she'd start to see herself through my eyes. I told her she could wear those pants to family gatherings where she played with her nieces and nephews. She could run to the store in them. "How about you take them home and just try them on again there? You can always bring them back," I urged.

Do you know that those red pants ended up being her favorites? She wore them everywhere! They added something to her wardrobe that was missing—spunk, fun, adventure. She loved them!

> ### DIVA SENSE
>
> "When I heard my daughter, at the age of ten, say 'I've got to lose weight,' that's when I stopped saying anything about losing my own weight. It worked. She stopped talking about dieting and being fat. I still think about mine, but I don't talk about it." *Pamela*

Shape Shifting

✦✦✦

I always thought that poor body self-image was something that afflicted only young women. Then I had the opportunity to speak to a group of women who were in their seventies, eighties, and beyond. I thought I'd hear their wisdom about how they stopped wishing for a different body. I was wrong! They were still dealing with the same issues they'd dealt with in their earlier decades. I had to educate them the same way I'm educating you. So don't wait another minute. Figure this out now so you can enjoy future decades without fretting over your shape. The right time to get right with your body is right now.

Although body parts seem to shift over time, not everyone gains weight or adds girth. Some people go down a few sizes after the age of fifty. If you fall in this category, it's important to realize that you may still be dressing for the size you used to be. You might be shopping for the pant shape you've always worn, when you could be looking at new options if, for instance, a wide bottom and thick thighs have disappeared. A good salesperson will help you get the best fit for a new body shape if you're still getting used to the new you. Any time there's been a shift greater than two sizes, get a helping hand. You need to be able to see your shape objectively.

Just as you're going to be dressing in hues that work for your particular coloring, you're going to be dressing the body you are currently in. You're over forty. One thing we know for sure is that you're not in a girl's body anymore, right? Seems like a simple thing to say, but lots of women don't understand where they should be shopping for clothes to fit them. Here are some of the major reasons women have problems with fit:

1. They are in the wrong size. Comfort and happiness could be one size bigger. Instead of going up a size, some women make adjustments to a bigger body by wearing clothes that cover their shape altogether, which makes them look larger than they are. Others may wear their clothes too tight, which also makes them look bigger.

2. They are looking for the right fit in the wrong department. Junior sizes are cut for girls that aren't fully developed yet, so unless you have a girl's body, you shouldn't be trying to fit into brands that are made for teenagers. Junior sizes are cut smaller than missy sizes, and missy sizes are cut smaller than women's sizes.

3. Sizes aren't standard; they can vary from one label to another, and from one store to another. If you freak out over numbers, you're more inclined to choose the wrong size. Fit is what's important. Forget the numbers on the hang tags and find the clothes that your body loves to be in. Life is sweeter that way.

4. Manufacturers make their clothes based on a fit model who may not be anywhere near your proportions. Okay, let's deal with it. If you have a body with a small waist and wider hips, stop complaining about not finding pants that fit. You need to go one step further: have someone take the waist in. No big deal. Adjust. It's that whole take-an-umbrella-because-it's-supposed-to-rain thing. You can be comfortable no matter what the conditions; you just need to adapt to them. I'd like you to do it with a smile on your face.

I've got a Diva Advisor here to help us with fit. She's a fit specialist. Her name is Catherine Schuller. She's been a plus-size model, has written for magazines about plus sizes, and travels all over the country educating women about their bodies and the clothes that will love their shape. (To learn more about Catherine, see page 94.) Even though you may not be a plus size, read on. Nearly all of her tips apply to any size. Then we'll discuss underwear and foundations. After that, we'll tackle problems you may be having with fit. Fit solutions will replace fit problems. Once that's handled, you'll be closer to that starring role in CSF.

Misfits

✦ ✦ ✦

There's nothing that makes us crankier than clothes that don't fit properly. It can ruin your whole day if you're constantly pulling at something. Clothes shouldn't be getting your attention. Your fans and your fun life should. Starting from the layer closest to your skin—your underwear—we'll review your body and fit issues from head to toe. Remember, a bad fit makes you look and feel bad. You want neither of those things. You're doing well! I know this is tough, but freedom from age-old issues may be paragraphs away. Hang in there.

Bras and Underwear

✦ ✦ ✦

More likely than not, you are in the wrong-sized underwear. Women's bodies change, and yet they continue to renew their subscription to the same bras and panties they've been wearing for years. We all know those guys who boast about wearing the same belt size they wore in high school, meanwhile, their bellies are hanging over the belt instead of behind it. Women are guilty of the same sort of denial. Ill-fitting undergarments will make for ill-fitting clothing every time. This week, go to a lingerie shop or a foundations department where a human being can measure you for a bra that fits you properly.

I was in the dressing room with sixty-nine-year-old Kate. We had been shopping for clothes, but I noticed

that her bra was doing nothing for her. "When was the last time you were fitted for a bra?" I asked her. "High school?" she replied. We shopped for new bras. Her bra size had changed from a 34B to a 32D. She was thrilled to be in the correct size. "This might have changed my whole life!" she exclaimed.

Here are some other tips on getting the right fit:

1. Consider new types of underwear. There may be styles you never thought about trying. Make it an expedition, a fun one. You may have worn a size 5 panty in high school. Don't be surprised if a size 7 fits better now. There's nothing to be gained by wearing a smaller size in anything! But too tight underwear, in particular, is a prescription for grumpiness, and a grumpy diva is not a pretty sight. Do everything you can to avoid the dreaded visible panty lines. They are caused by the following conditions: panties are too tight, the pants or skirt is too tight, the pants or skirt fabric is too thin, or all of the above.

2. Believe it or not, thong underwear may be in your future. It's perfect to wear under light-colored pants (nothing's dowdier than floral full briefs under white knit pants). It will also eliminate panty lines on close-fitting or light-colored pants. Dismiss any doubts

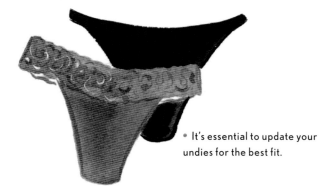

• It's essential to update your undies for the best fit.

HOW TO FLATTER YOUR SHAPE

· · · · · · · · · ·

BY *Catherine Schuller*

✦

Catherine Schuller is an actress, model, spokesperson, author, promoter, and marketer. Her goal is to change the world's perception of the full-figured woman.

1. Show more shape than flesh. A sexy silhouette accomplishes much more than exposing too much skin. Revealing too much flesh is distracting and destroys the mystery of the curve. We've been taught that revealing skin is sexy. It really isn't. Revealing shape is sexy.

2. Know your shape. Don't be a bud vase hiding inside a refrigerator box. Wear clothes that skim over your curves. Try a stretch velvet top, a wrap blouse, shaped shirt, or even a stretchy tank. The important curve is often right under the bust, so feature it every chance you get. Then add a layering piece such as a great jacket, shawl, or open tunic.

3. If you have a pronounced tummy or flesh roll at the side of the midriff (or both), steer clear of tops in fabrics that hug. Stick with a shaped, princess-seamed shirt in stretch cotton or something that eases over that area rather than clinging. Go up a size if you need to in order to prevent button gaping.

4. A smooth curve is better than a bumpy one. New technology in manufacturing shapewear has made it easier to get a smooth line from under the bustline clear to the ankles. Celebrities are all wearing these products to ensure an unbroken contour. The demonic VPL (visible panty line) is avoided, too, which is worse than chipped nail polish in my book! Getting in to the old shapewear, such as those heavy girdles, was like wrestling an alligator. Not anymore. New products glide on and even wick away perspiration. You can even layer shapewear for more confident coverage. You can wear a hi-Capri shaper, and than add a waist cincher. Or wear a midthigh shaper over a high-waisted legging style to give you a slimmer, firmer line with no jiggles.

5. Lift that bustline. Women often say they are short waisted when in reality they are low busted. Wear a great bra that lifts and separates. It's a must-have investment. You can then wear blouses and tops with darts and princess seams that complement a properly supported bustline.

6. Rediscover your waistline. If you've lost your waistline, wear a shaped shirt with some spandex in it. The shirt will find the curves under the bust, at the sides, and at the back of the body. If you have a tummy, it will glide over it. A V-neck opening creates a diagonal line, which, in contrast to the curves of the body, is very flattering. Flip the collar up, add a great necklace, slip into a fabulous pair of pants, and you'll look great. Be sure to wear it out! Your mother's voice, admonishing you to "tuck in your shirt," is difficult to forget. I love those shirts with the curved hemline instead of a straight one. They help to hide a tummy, elongate the torso, and look classic.

7. Instead of asking "Does this make me look fat?" look for good balance and proportion in the outfit. If you're curvier in the hips, balance your overall silhouette with an A-line skirt or one with a flared hem. If your silhouette goes from a wide hip down a tapered leg to the ankle, the contrast of too wide over too thin will make you look disproportionate and imbalanced, like an apple balancing on a pencil point.

about wearing them at your age and try them. Look for ones with really soft mesh stretchy fabrics. After wearing them for a week, you'll never look back. They solve so many fit problems. It's never too late to meet new underwear that's right for you.

3. Shapers, today's version of girdles, are essential to have in your foundations wardrobe. Yes, I did say foundations wardrobe. A great fit in a dress, pant, skirt, or top may be just a shaper away. Get a salesperson on your side and she'll help you navigate the growing number of choices out there, which are designed to give you a smoother line so your clothes lie better on your body. There are shapers available for nearly every body region—midriff, waist, thighs, calves, or all of those areas at once. For not a lot of money, you can look nipped and tucked without ever coming face-to-face with an anesthesiologist.

Details about Fit

✦ ✦ ✦

Now that you've put a date on your calendar to go update your underwear (you did that, right?), let's talk about other fit factors. Sometimes the body parts you used to highlight seem to have disappeared, like the waist, and you're left wondering how to dress yourself after all those years of tucking shirts into pants and cinching them with a belt. Décolleté is not as flattering as it used to be. Dressing with illusion might be a better approach than full disclosure. Not to worry. Confident divas work through fit issues, especially when their bodies have shifted weight or changed sizes. I'm going to show you how to look at your body objectively and

highlight your assets while downplaying any imperfections. It's a matter of making proper clothing selections and minor adjustments to proportion and balance. So you see? Even if this is a scary topic, there are plenty of solutions. The head-to-toe guide that follows addresses all sorts of fit issues. Find the ones you've been concerned about.

Take notes as you go and then make a list of things you're going to experiment with to free yourself of misfits. This list is one you'll take with you to your closet and on your next shopping trip. It's your research and development toward having a wardrobe that fits in all the right ways.

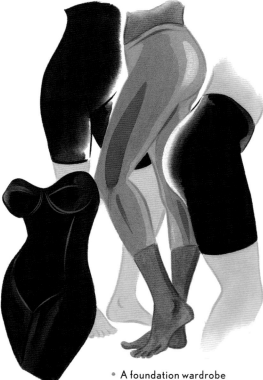

• A foundation wardrobe makes it easy to wear your favorite pieces with confidence.

Shoulders

+ ✦ +

If our shoulders droop, we look droopy and sad.
If they look too narrow, we appear less powerful,
and perhaps shriveled and old looking. Ideally, our
shoulders balance our hips.

1.   Create a straight line with structured jackets or
blouses. If you have sloping shoulders, be sure to add
small pads to square off your shoulder line and
balance your hips. (Avoid wearing them
under sheer fabrics, though.) Pads should
be invisible. Stay away from raglan
sleeves, which will make your shoulders
look smaller and more sloping.

2.   On the other hand, you might have
some jackets in your closet that are too broad or
padded. Have the shoulders reworked to create a
softer, more natural line.

• A jacket with a
structured shoulder
line evens out sloping
shoulders.

Neck

✦ ✦ ✦

As we age, we lose elasticity in the skin on our neck, so giving that area extra care is worth our attention.

1.   Try turtlenecks in fine-gauge cotton, wool, or silk to cover a crinkled neck. Caution: Don't wear a turtleneck that's too tight against the neck. When you move your head, your skin will be pinched and look more crinkly than it is. Go up a size if you need to and alter the body of the turtleneck. Even knits and sweaters can be altered.

2.   Wear a blouse with a substantial collar that you can flip up if you want. By adding a bold necklace inside the collar, you'll have some visual interest. Or try layering several necklaces together.

3.   Try wrapping a long oblong scarf around your neck, leaving the ends long in front or in back of your body. This is a lovely way to create beauty at the neck.

Arms

✦ ✦ ✦

If you're wondering if you can still show your arms, you probably can. If you're sure you can't, you might be right. Some women have naturally athletic bodies with strong arms, and they are lucky enough to wear sleeveless tops well for decades. But for others, even weight training doesn't seem to give a smooth look to the upper arm.

1.   If you're uncomfortable going sleeveless, be on the lookout for tops that offer the illusion of bare arms. These tops are especially good for evening wear or for wearing in hot weather. Look for stretchy fabrics made of netting. These sorts of sleeves will give you some bareness without revealing everything. A stretchy lace shirt with a woven collar and woven front plackets is a great find for creating modesty over the arms. There are so many beautiful fabrics available. Keep your eye out for luscious pieces that will give you coverage and confidence. It can be fun, like going on a treasure hunt.

2.   If a sheer sleeve isn't appropriate for the occasion, wear a sleeveless tank or camisole under an open shirt.

3.   Three-quarter sleeves are a lot cooler than long sleeves.

• Fabric with sheer sleeves give the impression of bare skin without having to bare all.

Bustline

✦ ✦ ✦

Whatever you do, avoid looking as if your boobs are ready to pop out of your top at any moment. There is nothing sexy about it. See page 82 about that proper bra fit! A demicup works for teenagers. You may need a fuller cup to give you the containment you need to create a smooth line.

1. Don't let your bra straps show. That was a Madonna thing in the '80s. Are you Madonna? No. Okay, so don't do it. If you're wearing something that might reveal bra straps and you wear a smaller cup, you can find bras with plastic straps, which are less conspicuous. Still, some part of clothing should be covering that plastic. Or wear a camisole or tank over the bra or a camisole with a built-in bra (again, if you're in a smaller cup). Then add another layer — a top that is filmy, sheer, or made of netting so it's still somewhat see-through. You'll get the look of bareness, but it will be more of an illusion. Very sexy. If you're larger busted, wear a tank over your bra (and bra straps); then add the second layer that is more sheer. Wearing a tank in a skin tone underneath a sheer top will give you a sense of bareness if that's what you're after.

2. If you're large busted, look for bras with fuller cups that will hold your entire bust and make your bustline smooth. Then be sure to avoid clothes that are too clingy, which accentuates the fullness of your bust and may throw off the proportions of your figure. If you want to show off your bust, that's fine. Just be sure to get a great fit when buying a top, so you look classy, not trashy.

3. A T-shirt bra is a must for wearing knit tops or tops made of thin fabrics, including shiny silks. They have a formed cup that guarantees smoothness. You don't want the seams or the lace of a bra to show through to the front of your clothing. Again, that's not sexy or cool. Remember, undergarments are not meant to be seen. They are just there to support your outer garments.

4. A woman's breasts and the curves that come with them are sensual and attractive, and they deserve a pretty line. If you're concerned about poky nipples, there are attachable, flower–shaped products available that will go over your nipples and smooth them out. You can also wear double-layered fabrics to help reduce this focal point or wear a T-shirt bra with a thin padded layer. Don't freak out that you're wearing a padded bra. It's just smooth so you'll be smooth.

5. To add more shape and emphasis to your bustline, button your cardigan or your shirt (if you're wearing it like a jacket) just under the bust.

• A closed button just under your bustline creates a flattering line.

The Roll

✦ ✦ ✦

Even if your weight has stayed the same, a roll may suddenly appear between the bustline and the waist. No matter how much you work out, it seems to want to stay there.

1. Minimize that curve with body shapers. They will smooth your shape so clothing skims the body rather than hugging it. Every movie star who walks down the red carpet is in one or has it already built into her dress. Don't be fooled into thinking actors just naturally look like that. They have engineered help, and you can, too. It's really fun to look thinner in seconds. Visit the foundations department.

2. Try clothes with corsetlike construction. Your wedding gown may have had boning built into it to hold a smooth line. A top with multiple seams from the end of the shirt to the bustline can duplicate this effect.

3. Avoid fabrics that are too thin. They can't hide a roll and in fact, will accentuate it. A garment made from a thicker, tougher fabric, like a denim jacket, will hold you in. But don't forget, fabrics with spandex added will allow you to wear jackets or shirts close to the body. Clothes that show your shape are always more flattering than clothes that hide it.

4. Wear tops with double layers of fabric to camouflage the area. Stretchy fabrics in layers that crisscross across the front can also minimize that roll.

5. Ruching, or gathered fabric, is another natural way to camouflage a roll. Keep going up a size until you find the one that makes you feel confident and not self-conscious. Remember, the size never matters, but the fit does. Go for good fit.

6. Fabrics that have been crinkled, crushed, or pleated or are heavily textured in another way, like seersucker, have body that holds its own shape and will camouflage yours. These fabrics aren't meant to be smooth. Many of us aren't smooth. So that bit of crinkled texture lets us be who we are just fine.

Thick Waist

✦ ✦ ✦

Many women famous for having defined waistlines lose them sometime after age forty. Blame it on the hormones. There are many ways to get around a thick waistline that will make you feel pretty. Choose from these options:

1. Bypass the waist altogether and wear a tunic or another type of top designed to fall away from the body.

2. Layer jackets and tops so they create interest—not directly at the waistline, but lower or higher. It's okay for a shirt to be longer than a jacket by one to two inches. This creates interest.

3. Wear a very long jacket that goes past the thigh and ends near the knee. Bypass the waist altogether.

4. Create more interest at the bustline with tops that crisscross the bust, distracting attention from the waist. This is especially effective if the top and bottom are the same color.

Tummy

✦ ✦ ✦

If you have a tummy that you want to minimize, here are some ways to do it:

1. Avoid wearing high-waisted, belted pants. Wear pants that sit below the waist. Below your belly button is best. Cutting the length of the tummy area will make it seem smaller.

2. Tucking in your shirt will only accentuate the fullness of your tummy. Untuck the shirt, leave off the belt, and let the shirt glide over your tummy. If you have a defined waist, then be sure your shirt has shape to it, with seams going up to the bustline. Shirts with slits at the side seams create more ease over the tummy area.

3. Wear stronger fabrics over softer areas of your body to give your tummy some built-in control. Jeans that fit well are a friend to a rounded tummy, as are well-tailored pants in a moderately thick fabric.

4. Shapewear will also smooth out the tummy area. Sometimes layering shapewear will give you the results you want. See what Diva Advisor Catherine Schuller has to say about that (page 83).

5. Do not let your tops stop where you're at your fullest.

The Booty

✦ ✦ ✦

Jennifer Lopez and the media have done quite a lot to help women embrace their curvy derrieres. Here you'll find tips for both showing off the curves of a full booty or making it less prominent if you choose to, as well as tips for creating more of a booty if yours is less than ample.

To minimize:

1. If you have a defined waistline, wear a full skirt. The fullness will cover your booty and make it less pronounced.

2. Avoid straight, tight skirts that cup the booty. It's best to go up a size so the curve of the booty is apparent, but the line falls straight down rather than curving inward to your knees.

3. Wear a jacket that falls away from the waist in back. A jacket that hugs the waist makes your booty look fuller.

To maximize:

1. Wear a skirt with interesting tailoring meant to emphasize the bottom. Try a skirt in a fabric that's cut on the bias to accentuate the curve. Or try a clingy skirt made of a body-hugging fabric such as jersey knit. Flounces also add fullness to a flat bottom.

2. Wear a wrap blouse that ties in the back and gathers over the hips to add fullness to a flat bottom.

3. Wear pants that have prominent pocket details that will bring interest and depth to a flat booty.

Wide Hips and Full Thighs

✦ ✦ ✦

If the widest part of your body is your hips, you've probably been told you have a pear shape. It doesn't mean that your hips can't be your favorite assets. This just means your hips are fuller than your bust. Full hips often run with full thighs. Using proportion tips, you can create more balance in your silhouette if you'd like.

1. If the hip is wide, wear a flared pant leg to balance your silhouette. A skirt with flounces above the ankle will do the same thing. Stay away from tight, skinny-legged pants. These will make your hips look wide by comparison. Also, when wearing pants, be sure that the hem skims nearly the entire heel. The longer the pant leg, the longer your legs will appear.

2. If you're concerned about a full thigh, consider a jean that has a "wash" pattern down the center of it so there's some gradation in the denim. If you're starting with a dark jean, the center area will be slightly lighter. It's like adding contour to your cheeks. The darker edges will seem to disappear, making the thigh appear narrower.

3. Full or A-line skirts are great because they're wider in the same places you are.

4. Once you've flattered your bottom half with a good fit, use the top half of your body to create the interest in your outfit. Do this with color, prints, layers, or details that draw the eye upward.

• Draw attention to your top half (and away from thicker thighs) by wearing bold patterns on top.

Cellulite

✦ ✦ ✦

Cellulite is a texture on the skin that most of us aren't crazy about. I see a lot of nearly naked bodies in dressing rooms when I'm putting wardrobes together for women, and even thin women have cellulite. Thankfully, most fabrics can camouflage it. One just needs to be careful of thin fabrics and light ones. I've warned you!

1. Wearing fabrics that have body, like a sturdy cotton, a heavy jersey knit, or coarse linen, will eliminate any self-consciousness around this issue.

2. If you're going to wear thin knits or slinky fabrics, especially in lighter colors, consider proper shapewear to wear underneath them. Remember, smooth. No ripples.

Thick Calves or Ankles

✦ ✦ ✦

When one's calves or ankles are thicker they can seem to throw off the proportions of the body. You might be slim everywhere else but here. Many fashion solutions exist for this issue so that the line of your silhouette won't be affected at all.

1. Wear long pants. Capris will only draw attention to this area by ending at the thickest part of your lower leg.

2. Wear stretchy ankle boots. Even leather comes in stretch, which will do a better job of fitting a thick ankle.

Feet

✦ ✦ ✦

We need to take care of our precious feet. Because of the pain we endured for beauty when we were younger, some of us see an orthopedist now. No problem. It takes a little more hunting, but it's still possible to find a fashionable shoe that is comfortable if you look hard enough. Some feet can handle different heel heights, but finding comfort might take an extra product or two. It's worth it.

1. Don't be surprised to be in a new shoe size. Your foot may have gotten wider. This is natural. Just to be sure, have your foot size checked by a shoe person. You may have been tolerating discomfort unnecessarily because you just didn't think of this.

2. There are a lot of products that can make a shoe more comfortable to you, from half pads or cushions to full inserts. Ask in the shoe department; go to the hosiery department, where they have feet fixes; or visit a good drugstore to find solutions. If you are wearing high heels, you will be putting a lot of pressure on the ball of the foot. Be sure to insert a pad there, which will absorb the weight. Or, carry an extra pair of shoes with you. Changing shoes, especially if you have a ways to go to get to the parking garage, will keep you from experiencing feet hangover the next day. Take care of them today and they'll thank you tomorrow.

Diva Assets

✦ ✦ ✦

There, you've done it. You've taken an objective look at your figure and noted what sorts of changes you're going to make. Now on to the fun part—your assets.

It's time to look at your body and decide what you want to highlight. Women are so not generous when it comes to assessing their bodies, so please, be positive and stay clear of the critic in your head. Kind and loving thoughts only! Often it's hard for us to see ourselves, so if you have a friend who can do this with you, that would be great.

Choose three things about your body that you'd like to highlight. Consider your shoulders, arms, hands, torso, bust, legs, hips, thighs, calves, ankles, and feet. Did you see *belly button* on that list? No, because no matter how great your belly looks, you're not going to highlight your belly button in public. Show it off at the gym or in your bedroom.

Keep it to three. If you were to highlight every part of your body, there would be way too much going on. Your clothes would be speaking so loudly that no one would be able to zero in and see you. You need to choose so you can strategically add focus to those parts you'd like to show off. Pick your top three. Now add an alternate.

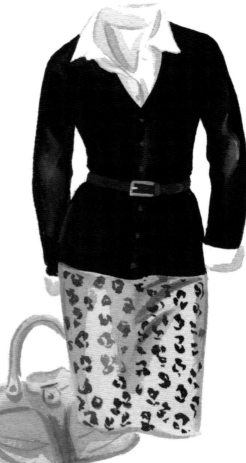

• Draw attention to great legs with a slim skirt.

1. ....

2. ....

3. ....

Alternate: ....

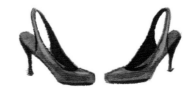

Now, just using your common sense and detective abilities, list some ways to naturally bring attention to those body parts. Look in magazines for people who appear to have the same assets as you. Or just look at pictures of those areas of the body in fashion magazines or catalogues, and see how those areas are dressed. Try pretending that you're advising someone else if it's too hard for you to think about enhancing your own assets. For instance, if a friend had great legs, you'd tell her to consider patterned pants, or pants with texture that draw attention to the leg. You might also suggest colorful pants or skirts, or slim skirts with details that attract attention. If someone were showing off a bustline, she might wear a crossover top or a colorful blouse with a pair of classic black pants so one notices the top area more. You get the picture. How will you focus attention on your body parts? Start collecting pictures from magazines that demonstrate great ways to bring focus to these areas. Then write at least fifteen ideas on a sheet of paper and put it in your binder.

Stand Tall, Be Proud
✦ ✦ ✦

A diva knows what to spotlight and what to camouflage. You may be worrying about your tummy when, meanwhile, someone across the room is admiring your legs and wishing she could have them. Remember that while you fret over some part of yourself. We rarely focus on what's right, I'm sorry to say, but doing so can make the things we're not as happy about recede into the background.

No matter what your assets are, practice standing tall. It enhances every figure type. Good posture is not only great for your body, but also lengthens it, making you taller and leaner. Practice good posture on your daily walks. Stretch your torso, put your shoulders back, and chin up. You'll feel two inches taller.

I think you're ready for your role in CSF. Open that closet door. Let's start putting color, style, and fit together.

DIVA SENSE

"I couldn't look at another pair of black pants. I had a closet full of them and not one of them was calling to me. I had a yearning for skirts. I don't think I'd worn one for maybe twenty years! I visited a friend who had just bought some skirts, and she was showing them to me. I tried them on and really liked them. So I went to the same store and bought three skirts. I had to get used to wearing a skirt again and seeing my legs, but I got over that pretty fast, and now I love it! Skirts make me feel more girly. They make me want to get out of the house."
Connie

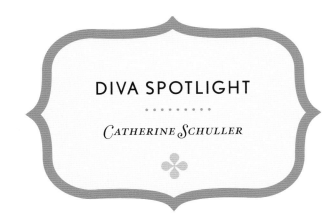

DIVA SPOTLIGHT

· · · · · · · · · ·

Catherine Schuller

✤

I am a die-hard New Yorker. I am constantly stimulated and invigorated by the energy in Manhattan. The Big Apple has taught me all my major life lessons and guided me to a self-knowledge and personal awareness I never would have found in another town.

What colors do you wear to flatter your natural coloring?

I am a natural blond, although I lighten and highlight it; who doesn't? I have light blue eyes and my skin tone is warm, fair. I wear autumn colors such as bronze, brick, and rust, and all sorts of shades of greens and aqua. I love warm and cool tones worn together because that mirrors what is happening with my hair, eyes, and skin. One of my favorite combinations is butter yellow and sea foam gray-green.

How do you flatter your assets?

Whether I'm in beachwear or dressing for the boardroom, I know what my assets are and I honor them, no matter what. I like my skin, eyes, and cheekbones and never leave the house without a good daytime makeup application: emphatic eyes, radiant blush, and a soft neutral lip. I like my bustline. Even though I am a plus gal, size 16/18W, I'm not overly busty (42C cup). So I can show off a little cleavage without it getting too risqué, and I always emphasize the curve under my bust to the rib cage. I have good arms from the elbow down and good legs from the knees down. So I wear a lot of bracelets and three-quarter length sleeves, and skirt hems that range from knee to ankle length. I always wear a slight heel to give that lift and sexiness to the ankle and foot.

Name a key diva piece.

A burnt-orange satin raincoat. I took it off the rack and thought, do I dare? On a rainy day I feel like there isn't a cloud in the sky. I wear it with a paisley brick-orange and black scarf in a lightweight wool. It's a classic look with punch.

What are your must-have accessories?

Your handbag should make a strong statement. Don't match it to your shoes. One of my favorites is a pouch with fur on the top and a long strap with a fur handle. I wear it with a simple beige Karl Lagerfeld coat. It's so outrageous. I also like novelty shoes.

An old favorite that you still wear?

I felt like I resurrected a friend I lost in high school when I had my tailor re-create a long Anne Klein blazer I bought in 1999. It's my power piece. When you wear a long blazer, it can be too blocky, but this one has high slits up the back, princess side seams, and three buttons high in front. It fits close to the body, is clean, has no patch pockets, and those slits allow a lot of movement when I walk. When I have to show up at 7:30 in the morning, I need a dramatic piece that helps me walk in and communicate that I know what I'm doing.

Name something you splurged on and never looked back.

I have a jacquard dahlia-print jacket lined in a leopard print — it's really a walking coat. It's got enough sheen to be dramatic for day, but it can move into nighttime as well. It was $800, and worth every penny. It's a substitute for a power blazer. The designer, Anna Scholz, printed on the hang tag "Dress to Devastate." That motto always comes to mind when I wear her clothes. How cool is that!

What's in your underwear drawer?

Comfortable, breathable shapers. Also underwear with a little Lycra power panel that holds me in. I am not a thong or bikini gal. For the most part I have lots of different types of bras: lacy, support, wild colors — all kinds of styles for lots of different tops.

Fashion rules you live by?

Don't go to the market in your sweats. Go dressed. You know you'll run into your ex! Image shouldn't matter, but it does.

Rules you break?

I don't have basic shoes. I never opt for "basic."

Do you have advice you'd like to pass on?

Just 'cause you can button it doesn't mean you should buy it!

BEAUTY SOAK With all this focus on fit, it's time to move your body around. This precious body that has brought you this far in life and has the capacity to keep bringing you pleasure desires some appreciation. One thing it loves to do is move and sweat. Pick an activity that you enjoy now or remember loving in the past — dancing, biking, walking, skipping, jumping rope, roller skating, or playing volleyball, badminton, or bocce ball. Make a date to do it alone or with a friend. While you are engaged in this activity, appreciate your body for all that it has done for you! When you get home, have a cup of tea, pull out your diva journal, and write a letter of appreciation to your body. I mean it. You complain about it a lot more than you bless it. Start making up for this imbalance today. You're about to try on clothes and get enormous pleasure from the things it likes to wear.

WEEK TWO

Chapter 8 • **TAMING THE CLOSET**
PAGE 98

Chapter 9 • **ACCESSORY NECESSITIES**
PAGE 108

Chapter 10 • **PUTTING IT TOGETHER**
PAGE 122

[Chapter 8]

✦ ✦ ✦

TAMING THE CLOSET

❋

I want to take a minute and remind you to look over chapters 12 and 13 ahead of time. See if you want to get some skin care appointments scheduled, or call this week to make your appointments for hair and makeup updates. Check your calendar to be sure you're on track for those beauty appointments you have planned and also for any predate details that need tending to. All set? Okay!

I promised you that the first part of Beauty Camp could be done in your jammies. The scene has been pretty relaxed, wouldn't you say? You've had lots of teatime to sort out your favorite looks, fabrics, and colors. Well, now it's time to get out of your jammies and get ready to jam! It's closet week! Get your supplies—protein snacks, your favorite beverages, and dance CDs. You're going to work! The next few days you'll be in your closet, turning it from a dowdy dungeon with too much stuff in it to a diva palace with key pieces that you love. We're on the hunt for CSF—color, style, and fit—that are right for you. Everything else is going buh-bye. I mean it. No more excuses for things that don't fit or flatter. By the time you're done, you'll feel ten pounds lighter, two inches taller, and five years younger. You're going to love that heady feeling of success when you've matched your color and style diva plan to what's in your closet.

Your closet has a lot to show you about what's working for you and what isn't. Once you've got the information, you'll be able to take it to the next level—completing outfits that you love and that love you back.

You're going to accomplish a few objectives in the next week. The first is to get rid of everything that does not flatter your coloring, enhance your style, or fit your body. The second is to discover the pieces that you really want to hold on to and work in to future outfits. And finally, you'll be on the lookout for support pieces that are in your closet—great-fitting things that support your star pieces. They could be black, brown, or camel pants; turtlenecks in different fabrics; or other good tops to wear under a jacket or inside an open shirt. Once you know what you have, then you can see what you still need. That will become your shopping list.

This might sound like a lot, but I'm going to break it down into very easy, manageable parts. At first you will be very active—trying things on, throwing some of them out, and asking yourself questions like, "What was I thinking?" I'd love for you to set aside a nice big chunk of time. So don't start this part at 9:30 at night if your bedtime is 10:45. Later, as we get into the chapter "Putting It Together" (page 122), you'll be playing with your clothes, which you can do in smaller chunks of time if you'd like.

Let's focus on the main goals in this chapter—the prep work for finding the ingredients you'll need for putting your outfits together. They're buried in your closet somewhere. It's your job today to find them!

Getting Started

✦ ✦ ✦

Turn off the phone, get away from your e-mail inbox, and plan to spend a few hours in your closet. Now, I wouldn't let you go there without support! I'm not mean like that. Gather your support team and bring it with you:

✦ Your resonance book, where you might have written things like "clutter-free living" or "wearing only what I love"; you know, the ideas or phrases you've been listening for that resonate for you

✦ Your Moving Away From and Moving Toward exercise

+ The pictures of colors or looks that you really love right now. If you put those pictures in your binder, bring that.

+ Your style words, which should be on a page in your binder or your diva journal

+ Your tic-tac-toe exercises

+ The boutique exercise results. Remember that boutique where all the clothing and accessories support you and your style?

+ Your beauty box for a restorative pause

Gather it all around you and spend a few minutes reviewing what you created last week. This is your blueprint. It's where you're headed.

You have three dates to dress for, but this investment in time is going to serve you well beyond those dates. It's going to set you up for success that will last a lifetime. Pretty high dividends, huh? So don't cheat yourself out of time for this phase. Review some of the tips Sunny and Gary Yates gave you for sticking to a project (see page 22) if you need help here.

Get some large garbage bags or some boxes for storing the items you edit from your closet. Don't worry about what you're going to do with the filled-up bags or boxes just yet. Keep a small notebook handy or use your diva journal for making lists with headings like these: "To Do," " To Alter," "To Shop For," "To Replace," "For Closet Organization."

Ideally, you're just looking at clothes for one season, either spring/summer or fall/winter. If it's summer where you are, and you have winter clothes in your closet, you can do one of two things: Move them out and deal with them next winter, or go ahead and review them *after* you're all done reviewing your summer things. Remember, this is a time-sensitive project. You've got dates to go on!

Feeling fortified? You should be! If or when you find yourself feeling bogged down during this next process, go back to your images and words and breathe them in.

DIVA SENSE

"Everyone told me that moving was a big job and I thought, what could be tough? It's just packing up boxes, right? Then I decided I would only move into my new home the things I absolutely loved. Being a recycler, I decided to 'gift' many of my well-loved-but-ready-to-move-beyond things to others. I quickly discovered that nobody else wanted most of my stuff either! I came to realize that our stuff — whether it's clothes, dishes, furniture, or cookbooks — is very personal. So as I'm shopping for new things for my new place, I'm feeling humble. I know to shop only for the things that I love, without any thought of passing anything on to anybody. We all have our own style. It's what makes us all so interesting and unique. That's why my motto is: Buy it, love it, but you can't take it with you and you can't give it away either, so enjoy."

Connie

Purge!

✦ ✦ ✦

Look inside your closet right now. I think it's safe to say you've got too much stuff. Coco Chanel said, "True elegance consists not in having a closet bursting with clothes, but rather in having a few well-chosen numbers in which one feels totally at ease."

If your clothes on hangers are pressing against each other, that's not good. Most closets hold clothes that are ten years past their expiration date. Let's get those spoilers out. What's making an exit today? Clothes that are out-of-date, dowdy, really old, don't fit, or aren't flattering because they aren't your color or style, and old favorites that were once brilliant but have lost their luster over time.

To make it easier for you, I've provided a list of items that may be lurking in your closet, ready to be purged. No dowdy clothes allowed in a diva's closet!

Items That Add Years, Pounds, or Are Not Age-Appropriate

✦ ✦ ✦

1. **Pull-up elastic-waist pants**, especially if you wear them with the elastic showing. They look like you've given up. If they are chic in every other way, keep them and cover up the elastic with something wonderful.

2. **White knit pants.** They show every single dimple and crinkle on a woman's butt and thighs. The white color seems to magnify skin texture. Whether you wear a size 4, 14, or 24, white knit pants are not your friend.

3. **Miniskirts.** Say your current age out loud and then the word *miniskirt*. Repeat until you lose your grip on the skirt and get a grip on reality. Miniskirts belong on girls and very young women. If you want to keep that black leather miniskirt, use it for bedroom costume play. It should never leave that room.

4. **Sweatpants**, especially if they are faded or if the seams, which once went straight down the sides of your legs, now swing around toward the front. These are so bad, you shouldn't even be sweating in them! A woman who respects herself doesn't wear these. If you have cashmere sweatpants in great condition, they are exempt.

5. **Warm-up suits.** You shouldn't be wearing clothes that so closely resemble a toddler's outfit—a pullover sweatshirt and pull-up pants with elastic at the waist and at the ankle. No.

6. **Jumpers.** These shapeless, long, and very full sleeveless things that go over a T-shirt are just not diva material. I know they're comfortable. So are muumuus, and those aren't okay either.

7. **Sweatshirts with writing on them** or with holiday motifs. If you teach preschool, you can hang on to one Halloween pullover. Otherwise, you're looking like a caricature, not a woman.

8. **Oversized sweaters** or your husband's shirts. Your clothes are going to fit your body and show your shape, not anyone else's.

9. **Suits from a job you had ten or fifteen years ago.** They're dated, they don't fit, and you wouldn't wear them to a job interview tomorrow or next month.

10. **Old formal wear.** Take a hard look at the formal wear you've been saving because it's too nice to throw out. Would you consider wearing any of those pieces on one of your dates? No? Then throw it out. It's taking up valuable closet space.

So, there's a start. You're looking for fashion culprits that are stealing away your beauty or not earning their keep. On the other hand, there may be some things you haven't worn in a year or more, but when you hold them in your arms, you fall in love all over again. Hang on to those. We'll play with them later.

Here's the strategy: Set a timer for half an hour and begin purging by looking for any items I've mentioned. When you find them, pull them out and start piling them on your bed or in a corner. Don't be surprised if a big mound of clothes rises quickly. This is good. Remember, you weren't wearing them anyway; they were just taking up space. All this old stuff doesn't hold good energy for you anymore. Don't defend these pieces. Let them go. Ready? Set? Purge!

Okay, time's up. You might have even gone beyond the ding of your timer. Great. It feels good, doesn't it? It's like losing the first five pounds on a diet. Easy. Do you want to take a break or are you on a roll? When you need to take a breather, sit with your beauty box and remind yourself of you. It will give you energy so you can go back and rid your closet of even more stuff.

I want you moving quickly at the beginning. Being around the clothes that aren't working for you can dampen your spirits. If you feel that happening, crank up the music, open the windows and doors for some fresh air, light a candle with a citrus scent (it's invigorating), or call a friend for moral support. Pretend I'm there with you, singing back your style words. When you defend something that's way off base, you'll hear me saying, "Dump it! Dump it!"

Set the timer for another half hour and get rid of the obvious things that don't fit. If you know you have clothes in your closet that are two sizes too big or too small, pull them out. If you truly believe that you'd buy those clothes again if they did fit, then put them aside and review them later in the day. This is a key question you're going to be asking yourself all day or all week, however long it takes to finish this job: "Would I buy it again?" And for you sneaky types, would you pay full price? Don't make any excuses or give any leeway to clothes you bought on sale. They need to meet your standards of CSF. This also holds true for the things you spent a fortune on and now know were mistakes. It hurts; I know it does. You can handle this. Purge for another half hour. If you find yourself slowing down and walking somewhere down memory lane, come back! Your diva style is waiting here for you.

Discovery

✦ ✦ ✦

After you've weeded out the dowdy and ill-fitting pieces, take a look at what's left. With the help of the color exercises you did earlier, you might find yourself saying, "Well, of course that's going! I so do not even like that color!" Or, "No wonder I never reached for that color! It makes me look sallow!" This is the time to remind yourself you don't need one in every color, just the colors that are good for you.

While you are weeding things out, you may come across the items that are just perfect for you. Start setting those aside at one end of your closet—all the things you love and would have in your personal boutique. We'll work with them later. Also set aside classic pieces that are in great condition. We'll use those when we're putting outfits together.

Look at what's left in your closet; it's time to start trying things on in front of a full-length mirror. You want to look and see if these items still fit and are in good shape. If you have the space in your dressing room or in an extra bedroom, you might invest in your own three-way mirror. Put that on your list (For Closet Organization) if it tempts you. For now, get a hand mirror so you can check out the back view of you in your clothes. If you try on things that don't fit well but you still love them, start an alterations pile. But be sure to ask yourself, "If it fit, would I buy it again?" Sometimes we just love things, but they aren't part of our future. Don't spend time and money altering something that really isn't diva-worthy.

Try on your pants, skirts, tops, blouses, sweaters, jackets, and shoes. Yes, shoes. I came across this quote by an anonymous person: "The best way to forget all your troubles is to wear tight shoes." It could be said about anything that's tight fitting. You can't possibly have anything else on your mind when you're in a skirt with a tight waistband or pants that are too short in the rise or are touching your thigh inappropriately.

Below are more signs of a bad fit:

✦ Cat-whisker creases in the crotch area of pants. (Usually not fixable, but a tailor might be able to let out an inch in the crotch to give more room.)

✦ Pants too short. (Usually not fixable.)

✦ Pants that drag on the floor (fixable) or rest too high on your instep when you have shoes on. (Fixable if the fabric will release the crease on the hem; take it to your drycleaners to test.)

✦ Tugging at buttonholes on jackets or blouses. (Might be fixable.)

✦ Waves of horizontal lines across the bust in sweaters or knit tops. (Not fixable unless the knit can be blocked by your drycleaner to yield an extra inch.)

- ✦ Sleeves that are too long (fixable).

- ✦ Shoulders too wide (fixable but expensive).

- ✦ Body of the garment doesn't relate to the lines of your body. (If you're tall and skinny and you choose pants that are made for someone with an hourglass figure, the excess fabric in the hips can be taken in, but if you're curvy and you choose a pant with straight lines, it can't be fixed.)

- ✦ Jackets too long in the body (often fixable).

- ✦ A waist that is too tight (fixable if the seam allowance is wide enough) or too loose (fixable).

Make some decisions about clothes that aren't fitting properly. Either commit to having them altered or let them go.

Diva Sense

"There is no end to the things that come close to satisfying but never truly satisfy. There are lots of brown T-shirts out there, but how many of them do I truly love? Maybe one or two. Those are the ones I'm keeping in my closet."   *Karen*

You're starting to see new life in your closet. Good for you! Isn't it amazing how hard it is to see what you've got when there's so much clutter in there? Now I realize that some people love getting rid of things almost more than anything. If you're that person, you're in heaven right now. And then there are other people for whom this is as hard as moving mud out of a flooded garage. If you're that person, easy does it. Break this into increments. Keep fortifying yourself by comparing your style exercises with the clothes in your closet. Look for a match. If *feminine* is one of your style words, which garments in your closet are feminine? If *sophisticated* is one of your words, do you have some clothes that are absolutely, undoubtedly sophisticated looking? If you're not finding matches, I bet you know in your heart what those pieces would look like. Make some notes in your journal. Shopping is in your future.

Next, go through the things you have in drawers. Review everything. Using the previous criteria, get rid of anything that doesn't work for you. Make sure that what remains fits and flatters you and is something you'd be proud to wear.

Next, get rid of the piles of clothes that are going out. Here are a few ideas for sending your clothes off to greener pastures:

1. Put them in your dumpster. The advantage to this is that it's just one step. You're done with these clothes. You've said goodbye. They are in such bad shape, it would be embarrassing to see them on another human being and totally not fair. No one should be wearing your trash. You might have some soft T-shirts that could be ripped up into rags, but you also don't need a sky-high column of rags taking up space in your garage. Be reasonable.

2. You can take things to someone else's dumpster, like Goodwill's. But honestly, don't make more of a problem for someone else. They get a lot of clothes, and many of them may better serve their customers than yours would. I know it's hard to get rid of things. Let this be a lesson to only buy and wear what you love. You'll need fewer things.

3. Give your better clothes to a women's organization that supplies clothes to women in need. There are wonderful organizations that help women get back into the workplace by helping them dress for interviews. But you need to be aware of some common-sense donating etiquette: They need clothes delivered in good condition — clean, mended, pressed, ready to go. If that means you have to take your clothes to be dry-cleaned or repaired before you donate them, you're looking at a few more steps to take. If they are contemporary styles, that would be a great thing to do. Otherwise, you might look at what you'd be spending to prepare your clothes and write them a check for that amount instead.

4. If you have a friend who fits in your clothing, consider a direct donation to her, especially if she's a mom who is too busy to shop or is between jobs and could really use the clothes. It's a win-win. But don't expect to give things to your friends or relatives thinking they will automatically love you for it. They may not want your old stuff either.

5. Mistakes that you made can be salvaged when you bring things to a consignment store but remember, they're only interested in taking the things they know will sell — good clothes in good condition.

6. Go online and find places that might need clothes right now. Unfortunately, there's likely to be a disaster somewhere in the world and organizations might be accepting used clothing to help others out.

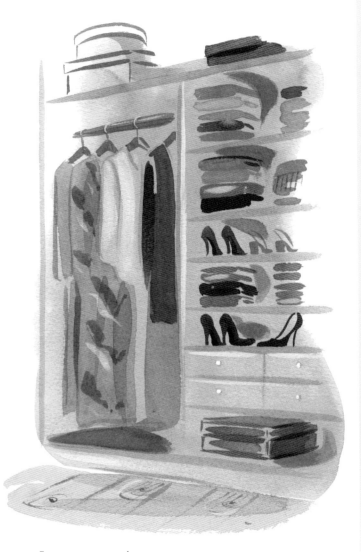

• For easy access and inspiration, arrange items neatly on open shelves whenever possible.

Assess

✦ ✦ ✦

Now that your closet is cleaned out, take a look at what's left. Everything that remains should be there because you love it, it's useful, and you'd buy it again, happily. You can use these things to create your style image.

Do your best to neaten up your closet, or sleep in the spare bedroom and handle it in the morning. In the last chapter, "Diva Forever," I'll give you ideas for organizing your closet in a way that satisfies you. Jump ahead to that chapter if you're on a roll and would like to perfect this shrine to your diva style. Remember, though, we have a lot more to do to get ready for your dates. You might want to conserve your energy, call it a day, and take a long bubble bath. Or rent a DVD. I recommend *Princess Diaries 2* with Anne Hathaway and Julie Andrews. There is a closet scene in that movie that is to die for! Believe me, you'll know it when you see it!

Next up is working with your accessories. Then we'll be putting some bundles of beauty together that will be the basis for your outfits. But you don't need to think about that right now. Give yourself a big hand! Sleep well tonight. You've done a fabulous job. With all that clutter gone from your closet and your life, you're getting closer and closer to completely surrounding yourself with beauty. This has been a huge step in that direction!

Let this be the turning point. From this day forward, you will satisfy yourself with beautiful things that fit your taste, suit your nature, and create joy specifically for you. Nothing enters your closet unless it does just that. Wear pink because you're crazy about it, stripes because you can't live without them, and lavender undies because in your mind, there just couldn't be another choice. Now have a good rest and meet me back here to go through your accessories. Those personal pieces are the glue for putting outfits together. I can't wait to see what we're going to discover!

Diva Sense

"You need to have clothes in your closet that you are totally in love with; it's as if you're having a love affair with them. Slowly I've been getting to that place. Why have clothes that you don't feel that way about?"
Jalyn

BEAUTY SOAK Get a cup of tea, find a comfortable chair, and browse through attractive magazines that you love, maybe on gardening, decorating, or cooking. Enjoy the colors, textures, graphics, and design. Continue to be a beauty tracker. Let your creativity flow into your surroundings. You might start a folder specifically for house ideas that have been stimulated by all your color and style work. Or you might want to take your creative juices and make a nice dinner. Give yourself time to enjoy the colors, textures, and smells. Then set the table in a style that relates to the clothing style you identified. Spread your style around the house, but just a little. Remember, no new big projects until Beauty Camp is over.

• Take a relaxing break to enjoy a stack of magazines.

Chapter 9

ACCESSORY NECESSITIES

Welcome back! I know you've been deep in your closet looking for CSF (color, style, and fit), and finding it, I hope. You've tried on your shoes and ditched the ones that don't fit, are too scuffed up, or are just plain dated. Now it's time to talk about the rest of your accessories—handbags, scarves, shawls, belts, sunglasses, hair ornaments, necklaces, watches, bracelets, earrings, rings, hosiery— all the parts of your wardrobe that don't need to be examined for fit per se, other than determining how well they work with your new look and style.

You do need to weed through your accessories (I'll show you how) and whittle your collection down to the things you love and that have your style words written all over them. If *dramatic* is one of your style words, but your necklace drawer contains nothing but thin gold chains that you never wear, you'll want to do some shopping soon. On the other hand, your accessories may be in colors you wear well, and can be described in words that reflect your evolving style. That would be a great beginning!

Accessories are multitaskers. They direct attention exactly where you want it. Want someone to notice your sparkly eyes? A sparkly earring on your ear—especially if it repeats your eye color—will lead the way. Want someone to enjoy the gorgeous color of your hair? Wear a scarf around your neck or a shawl over your shoulders that has your hair color in it, and it's all we can focus on. Have a waistline you're super proud of? A three-inch-wide belt will draw our eyes right to it.

An accessory can give you a power lift when it has a hidden message that only you know about. Jewelry may be designed with symbols that remind you of

what you'd like more of in your life—like devotion, tranquility, or wisdom. Wearing a necklace that has a pendant drop with the Sanskrit letters for *love* can put you in touch with matters of your heart. Jewelry that was worn by your ancestors can draw them near you even if they've passed on. Gemstones have attributes connected to them, so they can act as talismans. Scarves can bear images that resonate for you. The accessories you wear can be adornments of faith and strength.

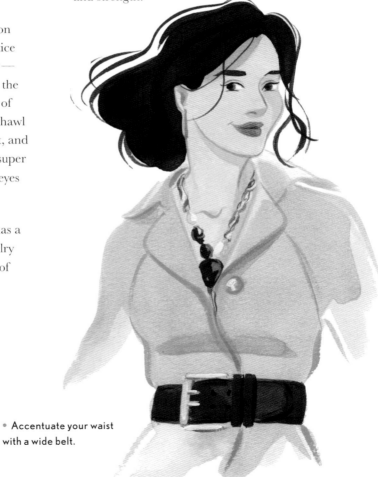

• Accentuate your waist with a wide belt.

Accessories as Infrastructure

✦ ✦ ✦

Accessories are also the infrastructure of a well-designed outfit. If you don't have it, your outfit will crumble. If you were to study a woman who looked fabulous and then mentally took away her accessories one by one, you'd see how undynamic she'd quickly become. Get your hands on the movie *The Devil Wears Prada*. Study the role accessories play in creating the put-together look of the impeccably dressed Meryl Streep, whose character is the editor of a fashion magazine called *Runway*.

Here are more compelling reasons to focus on accessorizing:

1. A woman who takes the time to put an outfit together and get the accessories right sends a strong message that she cares for and values herself. It's a great inspiration for other women of all ages.

2. Nothing makes you look fresher than a necklace and earrings that bring light and sparkle to the face. It can take ten years off your age.

3. Accessories make your outfits look richer, and when positioned correctly, they draw the eye up the body, which naturally makes you look slimmer.

4. Accessories that highlight your coloring and express your style will distinguish you from others who might wear clothes similar to yours.

5. Accessories are matchmakers. They are easy conversation openers for people to begin talking to one another. "Gee, that's a beautiful necklace." "Oh thanks!" And you're off.

You can't afford to ignore accessories. You may be someone who uses them minimally, but every diva, no matter what her style is, needs good ones to back up or create her diva look. I've got some simple steps to help you get your accessory stash in order and ready to play with. You're a pro at this, having done it already with your clothes.

1. Pull out all your jewelry pieces, whether you wear them or not. Go through them all and separate the absolute "yes" pieces from those that have little or no meaning or importance to you. Accessories are very personal. You might love the "yes" pieces because of their color, design, how they resonate for you, or whom they came from.

2. Separate any pieces that are broken. Put the ones you love in separate bags and plan to get them repaired. Some pieces may need alterations. Beads that are too long may be more dynamic if they rest closer to your face. This is an easy fix. Beads can be restrung and even redesigned using new colored beads or spacers that are more flattering to your coloring. For instance, a beaded necklace that incorporates your hair and eye color could be a truly valuable piece in your jewelry wardrobe.

3. Some jewelry pieces are classics, and we love them forever. Others may be dated and are just taking up precious space in jewelry drawers. Get those out.

4. Remove the pieces that have only sentimental value—like necklaces your kids or grandkids made you in school. Put these with other keepsakes, not where you store your jewelry. This storage area is precious and should be saved for your current wearable pieces only.

5. If you come across pieces that you love but haven't worn in a year or more, hang on to them. Fashion jewelry comes in and out of vogue. You may be inspired by something you see in a magazine six months from now, and that piece that has lain dormant will suddenly seem perfect. I have a long strand of Chinese carved coral beads that I keep because they're beautiful, although I still haven't figured out how to wear them. Maybe next year!

6. With everything weeded out and separated, group your jewelry by color, including metals. So if you have a lot of green pieces, separate them from the gold, the pearls and shells, and the coral, for example. If you have jewelry drawers, trays, or boxes, devote one to each color or metal. If you don't have these organization items, you might want to pick some up. You want your jewelry to be well organized, accessible, and also protected from damage or breakage, which happens if it's all thrown together in a drawer.

7. Now go through your scarves, shawls, handbags, sunglasses, hosiery, and belts. Put aside the ones you love or find useful and let go of those that don't ring a beauty note for you. Wimpy scarves will do nothing for a diva image. Nor will worn-out belts, dated or battered handbags, or ivory pantyhose. Let them go—into the trash, to a charity, or to friends. Get them out now. Arrange what remains on a shelf, in baskets, hanging in your closet, or in drawers so that you can see them easily.

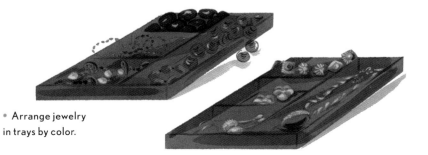

• Arrange jewelry in trays by color.

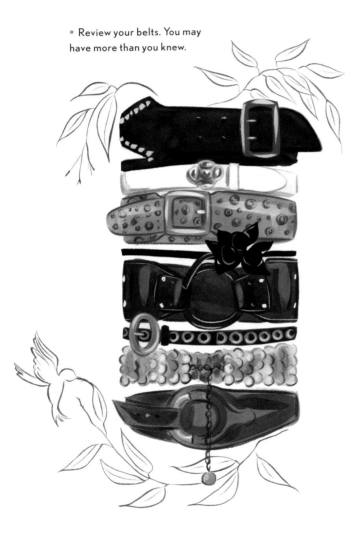

• Review your belts. You may have more than you knew.

Good job! You're doing great! Now you can see what you have to work with. You may have even rediscovered some things you'd forgotten all about. That's exciting! Make a note in your diva journal to complete an outfit or two using some of these favorite pieces. You might want to design a whole outfit around one of them in the next chapter.

Next, find a surface to work on—your bed, bedroom floor, or dining room table, for example. You're going to do something you've never done before. I think you'll want photographs of this next step, so if you have a camera, go grab it. These photographs will be great to keep in your wardrobe binder for reference later.

Choose one of the colors among your accessories. Now pick a place where you can gather all the accessory items in that color (several shades are fine)—handbags, shoes, necklaces, scarves, bracelets. If you have a gazillion pair of shoes in that color, then just bring out a few pairs. When you've finished with one color, go to another color and make a second pile. Work your way through the colors you have, including the metals, grouping metals in separate piles—bronze, copper, gold, silver, pewter. For instance, if you have a metallic silver shoe, put it with your silver jewelry and any silver bags or scarves that have a dominant silver look to them.

Take photos of these individual color groups. There will probably be some overlap. That's okay. Just rearrange your items as it makes sense to you and take more pictures. Terrific! These groupings should show you your accessory strengths, and the weaknesses, too!

Let's talk about how these accessory groups will work for you. Remember, they are the infrastructure of your outfits. Let me give you an example. If I was looking at my black group of accessories from my wardrobe, I'd see a satin crinkled scarf/shawl, suede mules, boots with heels, a beaded necklace with large textured and smooth lacquered beads, a multistrand onyx necklace from Thailand, a black belt with silver grommets, black crystal flower-shaped earrings, a small shoulder bag, a black-handled tote, and a jet black bracelet. I bought all of these items at different times, and I love them all. I could add any combination of them to pants and sweaters, skirts and jackets, and they would tie my outfit together no matter what color clothing I was wearing. From my feet to my waist to my neck to my ears, these black accessories would create a route up my body, connecting all the clothing pieces and tying everything together in between. These black accessories are the infrastructure of any number of outfits. I can get dressed quickly because these accessories are in place.

Recently I bought a high-heeled sandal in a burnished metallic bronze color. The decorative buckle across the front had an antique gold finish. It sat in the shoe box. I adored it! But it didn't go with anything. Sound familiar? I had introduced something in my wardrobe that was all alone in a color group. I took a shoe shopping with me and focused on creating a color group. I found a belt that had hardware on it in antique gold and bronze. Then I noticed a bronzed handbag with that antique trim on the outside pockets, which blended well with the shoe and a necklace of mixed metals. Suddenly, I was wearing that combo of accessories every day with different clothes. I wore them with a black skirt one day, white pants the next, and

jeans the day after. That group was tying everything together because the accessories related to one another in color and texture. It was as if I had all new clothes when it was really a group of accessories that changed and updated their look.

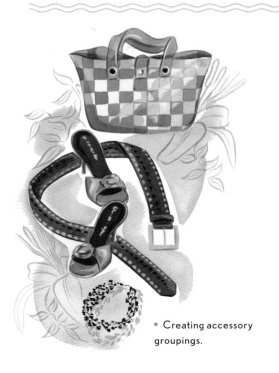

• Creating accessory groupings.

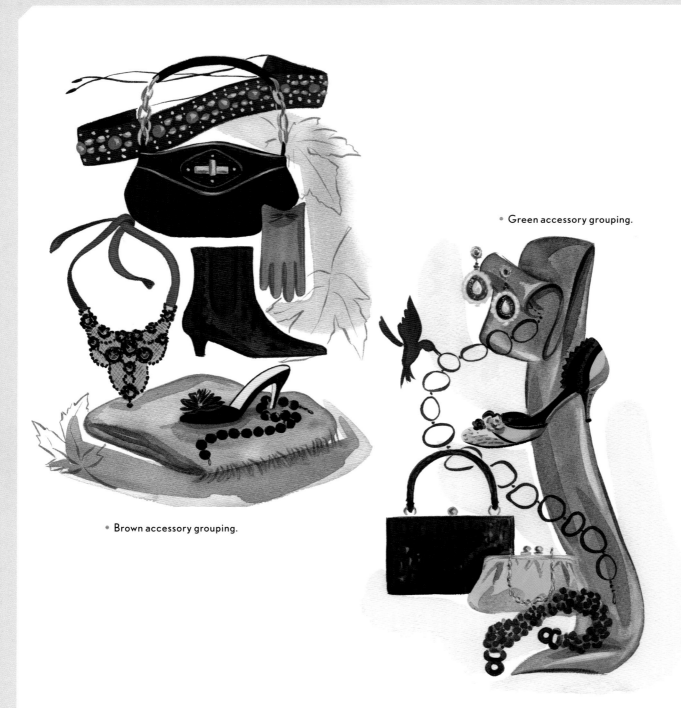

• Green accessory grouping.

• Brown accessory grouping.

Study your color groups. Do you see some that need developing? Do you have groups that relate to your skin, hair, or eye colors?

Think about hair color for a minute. Helena, who has dark brown hair, has dark chocolate pearls, heeled boots, and bags that look great with everything. Blond-haired Catherine has a tiered necklace in soft gold, another with blond wood discs, shoes in prints with a warm tan color in them, and bangles in shades that mimic her hair color. What do you have that mimics your coloring? Get out a piece of paper and write out a list of accessories that mimic your coloring. Check to see that you have some strong pieces in these colors.

Now look at your color groups to see whether you have a range of styles, from casual to dressy. Mixing dressy and casual pieces together can make your outfits much more interesting. A dressy handbag can make a casual outfit more special. A dressy shoe plus a dressy handbag will head an outfit toward black-tie. By building up choices within one color, you'll find it easy to put outfits together for all occasions.

I can see you! You're starting to understand why some things are so easy to wear and other times you really struggle to put an outfit together. If you notice some holes in your accessory wardrobe right now, start your shopping list. You might not find everything at once, but list all the things you'd like to have—it's a wish list.

DIVA SENSE

"My bracelets are all special. When one bracelet alone is too small, I cluster them in threes. I like to mix things. I mix a cuff with a beaded bracelet that has silver, pearls, crystal, mother of pearl, and wooden beads in it, and I add a charm bracelet. They all have a soft rose color in common, which is the color of my skin. I look at my wrist during the day and it makes me happy. It's so pretty. Because it goes with my coloring, it goes with everything, which makes it a better value."
Diane

If you've gotten this far and are asking me "What accessories?" you're in a great position. You'll start with a clean slate and get accessories that flatter your coloring or emphasize your style. Is there a metal that looks fabulous on you? Are there some pearlized colors that you love? Look at your eye color. Those green eyes would come alive in peridot, tourmaline, or green topaz earrings. A necklace in shades of blue would be fantastic with blue eyes. Pearls in the color of your brown eyes would be dynamic. You don't need accessories in a rainbow of colors unless you're someone who thrives on variety. You just need a few well-developed groups. I'll show you how to shop for these in the shopping chapter coming up.

I'm not suggesting that you always wear your accessories in one color at a time. That's just one option. But if you have at least one or two groups of accessories in a color or a metal, they will stretch your wardrobe like you wouldn't believe.

"I think as we get older, it's fun to wear bolder pieces. I wear big bold cuffs on my wrist. I have chocolate brown pearls that are long, and I can wrap them around my neck a few times. I'm wearing really big watches. I like statement necklaces, especially with luster or sheen. I have a textured chain necklace with sea island pearls, and every time I wear it I get compliments. The same with this chocolate crocheted beaded necklace. I like earrings that have a reflective quality. I want earrings with movement. Symmetrical tailored earrings that don't have movement seem too old lady to me now." *Helena*

Some accessories can work well alone, in accent colors. Dress elegantly in black or midnight navy and then add a golden sunshine–colored leather handbag. That can be big fun and a bonus, too, if your hips are a part of your body that you'd like to bring attention to (if that's where the handbag lands on you). Pops of color are like spotlights. If red is a color you've really wanted to bring into your life, a bold red necklace would do a lot to give you that boost of color energy. Or maybe a red silk flower pin, an arm of red bangles, or a red handbag.

When you are wearing accessories in neutral colors like white, taupe, khaki, olive green, brown, rust, black, or metallic, wear several for more impact. Creating volume can be dramatic and fun. Layering accessories—wearing two or three necklaces at once, two belts at once, or several bracelets on your arm— can be far more interesting than a single piece. Some divas, on the other hand, stick with a "less is more"

approach, preferring understated accessories. Understand yourself and let your instincts guide you.

Women make the mistake of thinking they have to find accessories to match every outfit. It's not true and, in fact, can end up looking as if they're trying too hard. If you try to match things too literally it can also look matronly. For example, avoid taking a color from a printed shirt and matching shoes, bag, and earrings exactly. When accessories match your personality or your coloring, they'll naturally tie all your outfits together.

Come meet Diva Advisor Cynthia Sliwa. She has a passion for brooches, especially vintage ones like those you may have in your own jewelry drawer. She'll share with you how to use this classic accessory with confidence and flair.

"For me I always go toward the elegant or the minimal. I don't pile too many things on top of that. I bought a red YSL bag and I got it in red as opposed to brown or black. It's a great accent to my neutrals. Because it has this organic shape, it will transcend the trends. Having a handbag you can wear forever is important." *Jalyn*

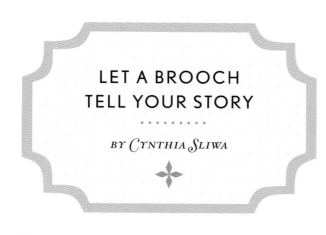

LET A BROOCH TELL YOUR STORY

· · · · · · · · ·

BY CYNTHIA SLIWA

✦

Cynthia Sliwa is an image counselor and the founder of Apprecia Fine Jewelry.

Brooches aren't just for Grandma any more! No accessory can do a better job of telling a story, while at the same time providing functionality and versatility.

1. Think of a brooch as a little snapshot of your personality, like a name tag but without any formality. What message would you like to send the world?

2. Larger, more unusual brooches can be great icebreakers, providing a ready opportunity for someone to strike up a conversation with you.

3. Brooches are easily worn in multiples. Collect compatible motifs, metals, colors, or shapes and mix them up for variety. Use pieces that have some unifying common element. Brooches are like punctuation marks — use them wherever you'd like to draw the eye. They're great on lapels and bodices to be sure, but can also add a delightful note to a shoulder, sleeve, waistline, décolletage, the back of a dress, or even on a hat, purse, or soft boot.

4. Wear your brooches in your hair. Use hairpins to fasten one (or more) into your hairdo, or attach a series of starburst brooches onto a ribbon and wear it woven into your hair.

5. Brooches can be functional, too. Use a large brooch to pin a shawl or scarf or to fasten a cardigan sweater.

6. Don't forget to pull out Grandma's jewels and give them new life! For inspiration, check out photos of the movie stars of the '30s, '40s, '50s, and '60s, who knew how to do glamour in a big way.

7. Finally, remember that brooches look great whatever your size and shape — the perfect pick-me-up for days when you're feeling less than your best.

A Few More Thoughts on Jewelry

✦ ✦ ✦

You may go through a period of several years where you wear a necklace every single day. And then, you may wake up one day and you're over it. That happens. Your attention may shift to some other accessory. You've entered a new stage. Go with it!

Some people invest thousands in fine jewelry, but then put it in a safe box and never bring it out. They're stuck with it forever—it was so expensive!—and yet they aren't wearing it. Then they feel guilty about buying other jewelry. If fine jewelry is something you keep but don't wear because it's not your style, give yourself permission to spend money on trendy, less expensive costume pieces and wear them with abandon. Accessorizing is about having fun. If something falls apart after a season, throw it away. You got your money's worth.

On the other hand, if you have great pieces that you're willing to wear, pull them out of the safe and put them on! If you have vintage pieces, that diamond brooch that was left to you by Aunt Helen, for instance, consider yourself lucky. Vintage pieces are standouts. The quality is usually fabulous and they're unique. Whether it's a brooch, a handbag, or a stole, pull it out and use it. These are little works of art, and art is to be appreciated, not buried.

To make jewelry personal and ensure that you're going to wear it, relate your accessories to the scale of your facial features. Look at your eyes, nose, mouth, eyebrows, and forehead. Are they small in scale, medium, or large? Try this. At a jewelry counter or even with your own jewelry, hold up a necklace that is similar in scale to your largest feature. Then hold up something that's smaller in scale. Do you see how the smaller piece doesn't relate at all? It makes no impression, while the item in the same scale relates so you see it. It looks like it belongs on you. I'll never forget the old Paloma Picasso print ads for her jewelry. Remember those big, chunky necklaces she wore in those ads? They were perfect for her because the scale was so similar to her features—full lips, big brown eyes, grand nose. She was a true diva! If you have small eyes, a medium nose, and large full lips, you've covered all the bases. You can mix scale all you like and it will work for you.

You can also mix different types of pieces. When I'm working with a client and am making outfits for her, I'll mix her accessories all up. For me the value of jewelry, belts, or handbags is not based on what they cost. I look for how well these accessories express and flatter my client. Don't be afraid to mix up your pieces. Fashion jewelry, costume jewelry, and even designer jewelry can be combined.

In the next chapter, we'll build on what you've been doing here with your accessories. We'll add some of your favorite clothing pieces and create what I call beauty bundles, things that work together and help you make outfits easily.

Can you see how things are all starting to come together? We have to take things apart, move them around, and help you see what you've got in a new way before we can combine them to make new creations. You've chosen your color palette, created your style words, and weeded out everything from your closet but the clothes you love or are useful. All the clutter is gone, gone, gone—miles and miles away from your house. (You did that, right?) You have a better sense of how to use accessories, and you know what you're working with for the moment.

Now I'd like you to meet a real diva in the accessory department. Gloria Untermann has helped my clients and me for years from behind the designer jewelry case at Saks Fifth Avenue. Her instincts and her eye are incredible when it comes to matching a woman to the jewelry that will make her light up with happiness. Her love for jewelry is infectious, and she's certainly famous for the way she wears her own. I hope she inspires you to reach deeper into your psyche to find what honors you.

DIVA SENSE

"Until this year, I never had earrings that moved. I only wore studs. Wearing an earring that moves is sexier. It makes me more approachable. When I used to wear my matching twin set and my pearl stud earrings and matching pearl bracelet and necklace it pretty much said I'm not approachable. And not much fun either. In all the time I've worn diamonds, pearls, or platinum, I've never had anyone comment on my jewelry. With my contemporary, good-looking costume jewelry, I've gotten compliments from men who never complimented me before." *Susan*

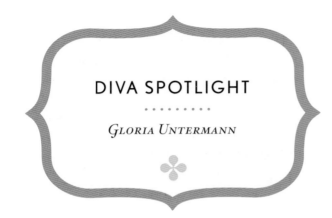

DIVA SPOTLIGHT

·········

Gloria Untermann

✤

Jewelry is my life! My passion for jewelry over a period of many years has given me a treasure trove of knowledge as well as opportunities for me to get to know some of the best designers in the industry. As a result, I'm in a position to help a woman understand how to achieve her own distinctive signature style through the proper selection of this important accessory. I think of personal adornment with jewelry as an art form.

What colors do you wear to flatter your natural coloring?

I almost always wear black as a canvas for the jewelry. The jewelry is always the focal point, not only for color but also to provide an overall statement of my personal style.

How do you flatter your assets?

By instinctively choosing diva pieces that complement and enhance those assets! I have fun indulging in what I have chosen as my signature style — bold, dramatic, unique, rare jewelry pieces or wearable art.

Name a key diva piece.

That's a hard to say; they're *all* key pieces to me! One piece that is unique for its type is a 100-inch strand of mixed jade beads. There's very little metal showing. It's primarily a jade story. I complement that with a pair of tricolor matching jade bangles, a jade ring, and a simple gold earring. Sometimes I add a substantial carved blue jade pendant for added drama. I would wear that while shopping in Hawaii. The idea is to feel free to "think outside the box" or "push the envelope" a little on every level. Have courage!

What are your must-have accessories?

For some people it's shoes, but for me, it's jewelry! Every day when I get up I ask myself, "What do I feel like wearing today? What do I feel like having on my body? What personal adornment do I connect with today?" Then I do a mental scan of my jewelry drawers. Do I feel like wearing turquoise, ivory, sterling, or gold? Do I want glass, wood, jade, or ivory beads? Do I want double strands, single, choker length, or long? Do I feel like contemporary amber or tribal amber? If I am feeling blue or tired, I choose something that will give me an energy boost. It's so intuitive. It happens unconsciously when I let my senses guide and inform me.

An old favorite that you still wear?

A jade ring that was custom-made for me by my dear friend Harry Fireside. It's always on my hand, and it's become a part of me now. I have many pieces of jewelry in my collection. Some I wear once a year or once every five years but each one is 100 percent right when I do — whether it's for a special event, work, a walk in the forest, or simply mailing a letter!

Name something you splurged on and never looked back.

My white gold Cartier watch with diamonds! Once a woman learns and understands how to honor herself and feels she deserves that special piece, decisions are simplified. When she acknowledges and respects herself, confidence appears and the previous barriers vanish.

What's in your underwear drawer?
More jewelry!

Fashion rules you live by?

I call it the 100 percent rule. Each piece of jewelry you consider adding to your accessory wardrobe should be 100 percent right for you. It's important to know how to select the right pieces for yourself. It's like a puzzle. If you become lost, confused, or bewildered, ask yourself what is it that you like or are attracted to when you stroll through a jewelry gallery. Do you respond to color, antique beads, retro pieces, contemporary art, or tribal art designs? You'll discover that you are more aware and in control of your jewelry style and signature than you might have realized. It's personal. It's powerful. Rather than being directed completely by trends, follow your heart. Have fun!

Rules you break?

Who says you have to *wear* jewelry? I enjoy living with my jewelry 24/7! I have a few favorite pieces on display, such as a basket of antique African ivory bangles, collectible antique Venetian beads framed as wall art, and strands of rare trade beads draped over sculptural pieces. For an unusual interior accent, I use interesting custom-made wooden boxes with glass viewing windows. I place wearable art pieces in the boxes, usually bracelets since they are my favorite accessory.

Do you have advice you'd like to pass on to others?

"Good enough" is not good enough. Each piece of jewelry you own must be 100 percent right for you so you can love it forever!

BEAUTY SOAK Make a list of things that nurture you and relax you — everything from taking a walk to looking through magazines, painting your toenails, doing crossword puzzles, arranging a vase of flowers. Try to come up with fifteen to twenty items. Write each item on a separate small piece of paper and then toss them all into a bowl or a box. When you need a pick-me-up, choose one of the pieces of paper from the bowl, open it up, and do what it says!

✦ ✦ ✦

Chapter 10

PUTTING IT TOGETHER

✳

Before we put together outfits for your dates, let's break down what goes into a put-together look. First of all, you know it when you see it. When someone's done it well, it's as easy to recognize as someone who's just fallen in love. There's a radiance about the person.

It's wonderful to behold women like this. It always stops me in my tracks. If I'm writing in a cafe and a put-together woman walks in, I can't help myself. I stop what I'm doing and I stare (discreetly). I want to soak in her beauty. It's magnetic. Even though I don't know this woman, I want to be around her! She's exuding a confidence and loveliness that is so inviting. Sometimes, I sit back and marvel at how she put everything together.

Keep your eyes open for these women; they're great teachers. Study what they're doing. It's usually a rich combination of CSF and an outfit that's made up of star pieces, support pieces, accessories, and the finished look that comes from a current hairstyle and polished makeup. When someone's look gets your attention, notice her jewelry, shoes, and color combination. Watch how your eyes travel around her outfit, taking it all in. What makes your eyes move from foot to head? The colors? The textures? The accessories? The way they blend together? Train yourself to come up with words to explain what's going on.

You're going to be one of those put-together women. You're going to be highlighting your assets, sharing aspects of yourself with others. You'll do it with the colors you choose, the clothes that speak to your style, and the finishing touches: your accessories, updated hairstyle, and makeup.

Put yourself in places where you might observe some pros. One place to feast your eyes on put-together women is at fashion shows in department stores or charity events, especially if the models are "real" women of various ages with real bodies. Get yourself to these if you can. Make them one of your beauty soak experiences. Even if the models are professional, you'll get a chance to see outfits that are really finished.

I've played a role in many of these fashion shows. As the guest speaker for the event, I often comment on the clothes. I'm there all day familiarizing myself with the merchandise that's being featured. Let me tell you about how these shows always inspire me.

Hours before the event, I'll be in a back room reviewing the "pull," which is what they call the selected outfits from the selling floor that are hanging on rolling racks all steamed and ready for the models who will be wearing them. Hanging with the outfits are all the accessories. The jewelry pieces are inside of bags, as are the sunglasses, headbands, and scarves. The handbag selected for an outfit is hung over a hanger. Beneath the outfit is the chosen shoe. It may be more expensive than any piece from the sponsoring department, but it won't be referenced in the show. The managers are selling you on the clothes from those departments, not the accessories from downstairs. But don't be fooled, without all those other pieces, the clothes would never look as good.

It takes thought and stuff — the right stuff — to create a great look. I'm going to help you figure out what you need to put your three date outfits together. With all of this practice, you'll soon be putting clothes together like a pro.

In order to put together your own outfit, you need the following three elements:

1.   You need star pieces — items in your wardrobe that stand out for one reason or another, like a Chinese kimono, an embroidered jacket, a butter-yellow leather jacket, pants made from a jacquard fabric that's attention getting on its own. These pieces aren't ordinary. There's something special and unique about them.

2.   Next you need support pieces — those pieces you can count on to support your star pieces. They generally are pants, skirts, blouses, and T-shirts that are pretty simple in design but of good quality. They step in at a moment's notice, support your star piece, and make it the focal point it wants to be.

3. Finally, you need some accessories you can count on that work well with one another and will tie your outfit together from head to toe.

If you're missing any of these key ingredients, you'll constantly feel as if you don't have anything to wear. You'll come up with excuses for not joining friends for fun events. I don't want this to happen to you!

Today you're going to find the star pieces in your closet that could work for your three dates. You're also going to identify any support pieces you have. You'll start putting together outfits by creating what I call beauty bundles, which are transitional steps. These are three or more items that work well together. They'll include a star piece of clothing plus a couple of accessories, which together will make up at least half of an ensemble. A beauty bundle is a stepping stone to confident dressing.

If you've got a good start, the finished outfit won't be far behind. It's sort of like having core ingredients in your refrigerator at the ready for when friends stop by unexpectedly. You know you will be able to confidently throw together some quick hors d'oeuvres, open a bottle of wine, and be a calm and gracious host, enjoying the company of your friends. I want you to have that same confidence with your clothes. When you identify a beauty bundle, write it down as you would a recipe. You won't store your beauty bundles together in your closet, but you will be able to gather them any time you wish and put a terrific outfit together on the spot.

When you play with your clothes today, think of them as ingredients. A lot of times, you can mix things from your work wardrobe, like pin-striped pants or a simple blazer, with pieces that are for social occasions, for example frilly sheer tops and floral skirts. Don't be limited by the ways you wore them before.

Let's get back to your closet.

The ingredients for your three dates are either in this closet of yours or they're not, in which case you're going to go shopping. If the word *shopping* makes you grab your wallet and coat and race ecstatically to the door, stop! Hold on to your panties and your wallet! It's not time yet. I'll blow the shopping whistle when it is.

• Classy work pants make an excellent support piece for a feminine blouse.

If you're the kind of person who'd rather lay bathroom tile or hang wallpaper than go clothes shopping, you're getting a reprieve—for now. You don't have to face those dressing room mirrors under bad lighting or get bombarded by styles that make you cringe. Don't worry. I've got shopping strategies that will transform the experience for you. It'll be as easy as tic-tac-toe (hint, hint). For now, you're going shopping in your closet.

This is playtime. I hope you've got a chunk of time before you. It is a creative process, so don't rush through it. Slow down, take deep breaths. Let me hear those exhales! You've done so much to be ready for this step. You've got your CSF handled. Now, whether you're an extroverted life-of-the-party person or a quiet introvert who loves to hang out alone near burbling creeks, your diva DNA begs to be honored. Let's see if it's there in your closet.

While you're playing around in your closet, you may find yourself putting together way more than three outfits. Great! Just promise me this: Record them. Write them down so you have a lasting image of them. Or photograph them. Believe me, when the creative juices are flowing, you'll look in the mirror and say to yourself, "I'll never forget this. It's so darn cute!" It is, but you will forget how you did it. By next Tuesday, you'll be trying to figure out what went with what. You can use the simple format on the following pages to record your outfits, so copy it and keep the blanks in your wardrobe binder. Fill them out whenever you get time to play in your closet and make new outfits. Add the key style words that are being expressed in this outfit. It's good practice to keep seeing your style words in your outfits.

•• Outfits ••

Top:

....

....

Bottom:

....

Jacket:

....

Shoe:

....

Accessories:

....

Finishing details:

....

Where I'll wear this:

....

Key style words:

....

....

....

....

Top:

....

....

Bottom:

....

Jacket:

....

Shoe:

....

Accessories:

....

Finishing details:

....

Where I'll wear this:

....

Key style words:

....

....

....

....

Top:

Bottom:

Jacket:

Shoe:

Accessories:

Finishing details:

Where I'll wear this:

Key style words:

Top:

Bottom:

Jacket:

Shoe:

Accessories:

Finishing details:

Where I'll wear this:

Key style words:

Top: ....

....

Bottom: ....

....

Jacket: ....

....

Shoe: ....

....

Accessories: ....

....

Finishing details: ....

....

Where I'll wear this: ....

....

Key style words: ....

....

....

....

....

....

Top: ....

....

Bottom: ....

....

Jacket: ....

....

Shoe: ....

....

Accessories: ....

....

Finishing details: ....

....

Where I'll wear this: ....

....

Key style words: ....

....

....

....

....

....

Your Date

✦ ✦ ✦

To refresh your memory, one of your dates will be at home. You've probably decided whether it will be dressy or casual. Most likely you'll want to be comfortable, relaxed, yet glamorous in some way. You're the hostess! The other two dates are outside your home. One is casual, and the other more dressy. For those outside dates, you want to get dressed so you look and feel too cute to go home. (I stole that line from a bumper sticker.)

Star Pieces

✦ ✦ ✦

Let's start by identifying and pulling out your star pieces, the contenders for your date outfits. Go to your clean closet and pull out ten of them. They are great items because of the quality, some special detail, or maybe for the way they fit you so perfectly and show off one of your best assets. You can choose them from clothing items, shoes, jewelry, scarves—anything that you'd be excited to wear. Spread those ten items across your bed. Or, if you have a portable clothing rack, set it up and hang the items on that rack so you can see them outside your closet.

You notice I don't distinguish clothes from accessories when I talk about star pieces. When you're putting a look together, sometimes it's the accessory that excites you and calls out to be worn—a bold necklace,

a cheetah print high-heel pump, a sparkly handbag, an embroidered shawl. I want you to know your wardrobe so well that you can build outfits starting anywhere. What are your star pieces? List them on a sheet of paper.

DIVA SENSE

"I wore an outfit that I really liked for a New Year's gathering at my house. It was centered around this black velvet stretchy top with fur trim that tied under my bustline. I wore a satin black camisole underneath with a curved hem that I left untucked. It looked a little sexy and relaxed, and I felt adorable and fun with that fur framing my neck and plunging down, bringing attention to my chest, which I like. I had on wool pants, which I usually wear for work. I added open-toed, kitten-heeled sandals. The outfit was so comfortable, but as I said, really cute. I wanted to wear it again. So I hosted a birthday party for a friend the next month and asked everyone to come in dressy clothes — even though it was for lunch. We're a group of women who meet every month, always in jeans and T-shirts. Everyone dressed up! I hardly recognized my friends! We all felt so special, so grown-up and sophisticated. Dressing up made the day so lovely and memorable."

Connie

I asked a couple of divas to share their star pieces with you. Check them out. See if you can imagine how they look and why.

Jalyn's Star Pieces

✦ ✦ ✦

• Distressed-leather jacket
with a one-button closure in
the front that has a wavy and
asymmetrical raw edge all
around it.

• Ankle-wrapped, python-
printed platform sandals with
a rose garden motif stamped
into the leather covering the
platform.

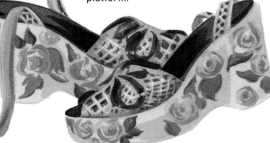

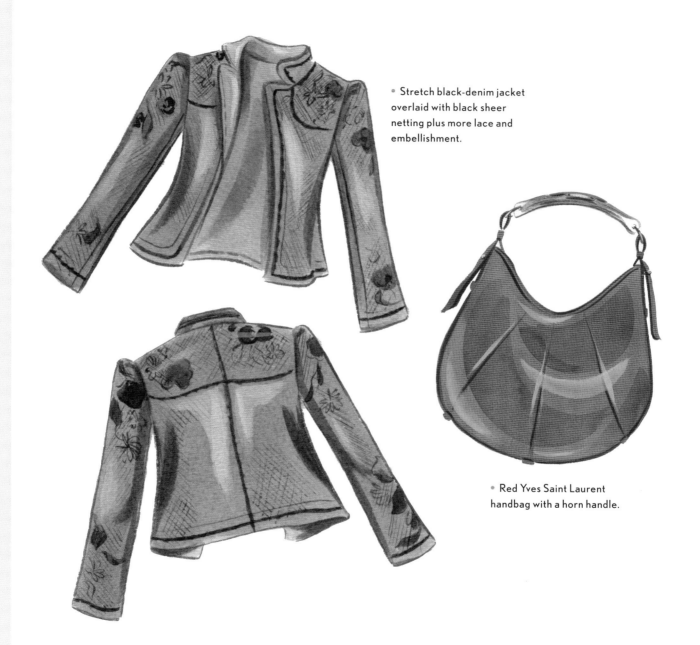

• Stretch black-denim jacket overlaid with black sheer netting plus more lace and embellishment.

• Red Yves Saint Laurent handbag with a horn handle.

Helena's Star Pieces

✦ ✦ ✦

• Burgundy suit with double rows of brown topstitching throughout, making it look contemporary and youthful.

• Long strand of chocolate brown pearls that can be wrapped several times around the neck.

• Bronzy metallic satin trench coat.

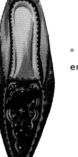

• Moroccan-style embroidered mules.

Supporting Roles

✦ ✦ ✦

An outfit is not all about the star piece. You need good support pieces, too. You need those sleek, simple pants to wear with that sexy, off-the-shoulder jersey knit wrap top. The top will be the star of the outfit, and everything will be there to enhance the impact of that alluring top. A strappy shoe that shows some bareness at the foot will add to the outfit's sexy quality. So will earrings with movement and sparkle, bringing attention to the face.

Support pieces need to be great on their own. If they are clothing, they're made from a quality fabric, are well cut, and fit really well. The better these pieces look, the better the star piece will look. Key support pieces are often T-shirts (short-sleeved, long-sleeved, sleeveless); cardigan sweaters or sweater sets; and V-neck sweaters or turtlenecks. They are also those boots that you can wear with everything, and a wrap that works well. They are simple pants—dressy, casual, or in between—plus jeans in different shades. Support pieces usually have few distinguishing details.

• Great support pieces . . .

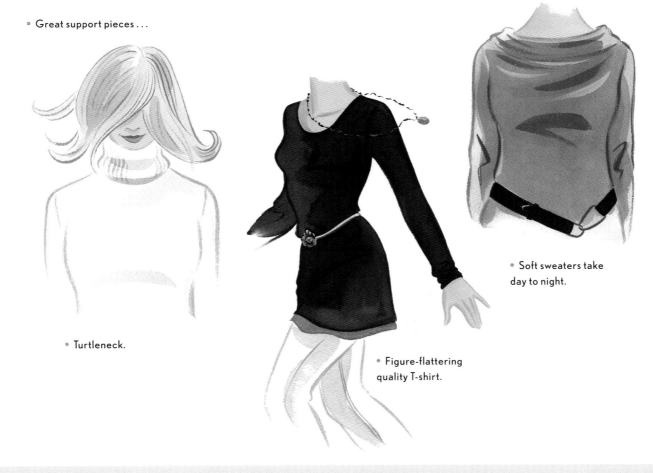

• Turtleneck.

• Figure-flattering quality T-shirt.

• Soft sweaters take day to night.

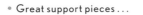
• Great support pieces . . .

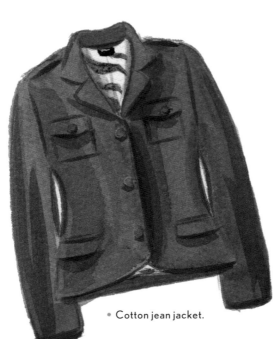
• Cotton jean jacket.

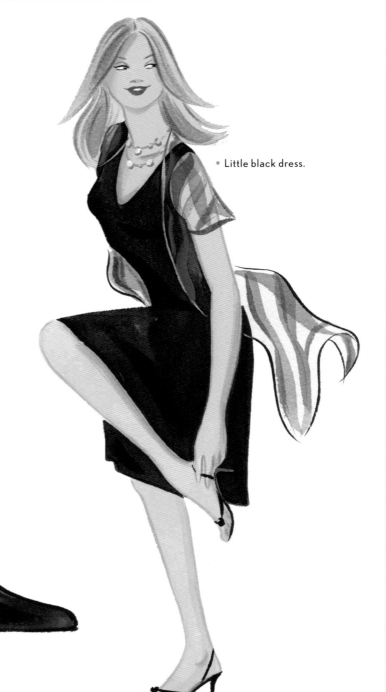
• Little black dress.

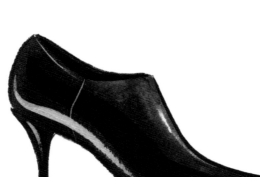
• Sleek ankle boot.

Helena's Support Pieces

✦ ✦ ✦

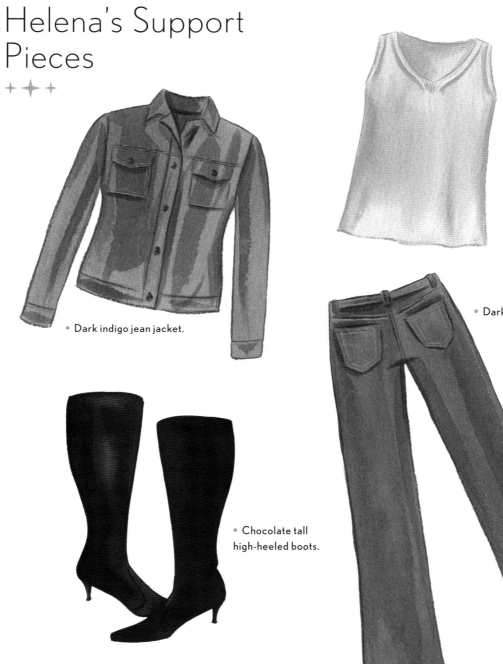

Dark indigo jean jacket.

Cashmere tank.

Dark indigo jeans.

Chocolate tall high-heeled boots.

Take a look through your closet and pull out your key support pieces. Put them on one end of your portable rack or the edge of your bed. Study their condition. They get a lot of wear—more than the star pieces.

When you've decided what your support pieces are, make a list of them. Keep a copy in your wallet. When you find yourself with some spare time for shopping, start looking to replace them now, before they are in bad shape and you're desperate.

My Key Support Pieces

✦ ✦ ✦

DIVA SENSE

"Every year I go out and buy new T-shirts. They are so important to my wardrobe and they get tattered after a year of heavy use. I freshen up my collection in my basic colors and styles — short-sleeved choices plus sleeveless for under jackets. They do a lot for making my outfits look great."   *Debra*

Support pieces need not be boring. While I was interviewing divas for this book, one thing that became clear was that even their basics had something special about them. The T-shirts were finely knit or a blend that made them smooth and dressier looking. The crossover tops were in velvet or a pretty netting fabric and in great colors, which made them more interesting. Boots had great detailing, even though they were simple. Jeans weren't ordinary. They were contemporary, well fitting, and a notch or two better than the average choices that were out there. If you're shopping for support pieces, make them special and of good quality. They'll make every outfit you put them with look that much better.

This brings me to a commonly asked question: "How many pairs of black pants does someone need, really?" If black pants are a key support piece and you generally make the top part of your body the star area, then you probably need several styles of pants that will take you from dressy to casual in your life. But here's a word of caution: One reason people may have so many pairs of black pants in their closet (or another clothing item) is that they never buy *the* one that truly is best. It's a funny thing. You can buy five white shirts that come close but aren't really the quality you want.

The one you want might cost more, and you deny yourself the pleasure of having it. Meanwhile, if you add up the cost of the ones you bought and don't wear or aren't really satisfied with, it probably exceeds the price of the one you really wanted in the first place. Go for satiation, not quantity. If this means I've just given you permission to get rid of those ten pair of pants that were "just okay," then you have more weeding to do in your closet. Continue to edit things as we go along. Better to have fewer things and really wear them.

What to Buy Twice

✦ ✦ ✦

Sometimes it's smart to buy doubles or triples of the same exact piece. If you find the perfect pair of pants, wouldn't it be smart to buy two of them so you can hem one of them for your highest heeled shoes and one for your lower shoes? One hem length will not work for all shoe heights. Those great pants that are the right length when worn with tall shoes will drag on the floor and look sloppy with lower shoes. You might wear one pair for a while before taking off the tag on its twin in case it doesn't end up working as well as you thought it would. Do this for jeans. When you find a great pair that works, buy two and hem them for different shoe heights. When you find the perfect shell or tank that is a mainstay for lots of different outerwear, buy more than one. If you're fuller in the bust and want to minimize attention in that area, you might be on the search for the perfect sweater that shows your shape without hugging too tightly. When you find this sweater, you might want two of them in different

colors (your best colors), but no more. I'm pressing this point because it really can make life so simple for you. I know we have a shopping chapter ahead, but it's good to be planning this now when you're in front of your closet and deciding the status of your pieces.

Sometimes a wardrobe is missing star pieces. This happens when women have played it safe and stuck to a practical plan with no passion. If you're missing star pieces you're really in love with, get them on your shopping list. I want you to have time to pick them up for your dates.

If your style is simple like our diva Debra Cox (see page 55), it might seem to you that most of your wardrobe is made up of support pieces. That's fine. If everything has a measure of quality, when you put it together, it will speak volumes about your sophistication and good taste.

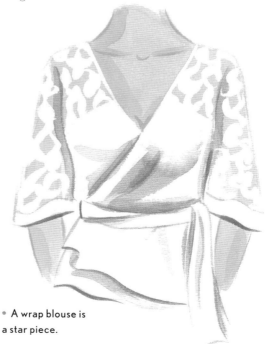

• A wrap blouse is a star piece.

"My secret weapon is my pair of flared black wool trousers, which never seem to wrinkle, are cut a little low so they're never tight on my waist, and can be worn year-round. For a dressy look, they're perfect with my black Chanel-style jacket with jet buttons, a sequined tank underneath, and open-toed sandals. They're fabulous with my zebra-print long jacket, white blouse, and black boots for daytime. They spiff up a T-shirt and jean jacket, which I wear with a fun scarf, for a casual dinner or party. I could wear them every day of the week and make them look different."

Connie

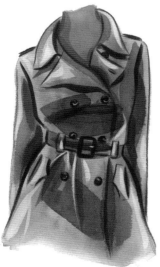

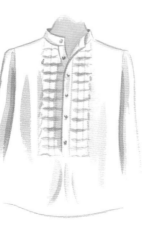

• A shiny trenchcoat and a ruffled blouse make classical pieces.

Building Beauty Bundles

✦ ✦ ✦

Okay, you've identified your star pieces and your support pieces. Let's start building a beauty bundle. Start with one of your star pieces. Make this one an article of clothing. Lay it on your bed. What is going on with it? Name the color or colors. Name the texture; is it shiny, smooth, nubby, sparkly, hard, soft? Is there a pattern to it? Is it a themed piece—like a jacket with Chinese characters on the back? What you're going to put with it can repeat one or more of these elements—color, texture, theme. Decide what two things, other than clothing, would go well with it. You'll need shoes and a handbag for sure, so see if you have those pieces. Do you have earrings that would go well with that piece? How about a belt, watch, or a scarf?

Let me give you examples of beauty bundles from my wardrobe. One of my star pieces is a nutmeg-colored, soft wool outer coat that comes to my knees—pretty classic except for the attached hood. The coat is lined in the same nutmeg color, only in satin. The hood gives it a sporty feel, the satin gives it a glamorous quality, and both of those words came out of my style exercises. The coat has slit pockets in front and gorgeous buttons, which I put on myself because I didn't like the ones that came with it. I usually wear it open and unbuttoned. Four other things look great with this coat:

1. Caramel-colored double strand of pearls.

2. Nutmeg-colored suede boots.

3. Leather clutch bag in a caramel-brown shimmery color. It's encrusted with big matching colored gems on the front of it, which make it sparkle like crazy.

4. Suede hobo bag the same color as the coat.

When I lay these pieces on the bed together, I just swoon with delight. They are definitely a bundle of beauty. To put outfits together with this nutmeg beauty bundle, I only need to add a top and a bottom. For a casual chic look, I've worn a dressy, flared-leg pair of jeans with it and added a black crossover sweater. I wear a hobo bag during the day, the gemstone bag

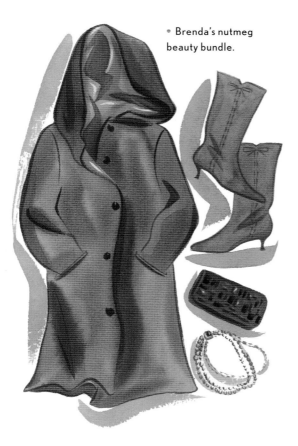

• Brenda's nutmeg beauty bundle.

at night. The repeated nutmeg color and the pearls pull in the highlights in my hair. I look instantly put together. I've also worn a simple black crew-neck sweater and a pair of ivory silk-and-wool pants under that coat and kept the same boots and the pearls.

Let me share with you another beauty bundle of mine. This one focuses on the color black. You'll recognize some of these pieces because they're in my black accessory group:

1. Black jacket, dressy looking with a floral black-on-black satin print, shiny black beaded buttons, and little slits—two on the front, two on the back.

2. Satin long rectangular crinkle-pleated black scarf, which can be wide like a shawl or gathered and tied as a scarf.

3. Black crystal earrings shaped like roses.

4. Necklace of large black beads, which resemble pearls, mixed with beads covered in black ribbons. It ties with a ribbon behind my neck, so I can adjust the length.

5. Small oblong smooth black leather handbag with little leather laces tied in bows at the corners and two short shoulder straps in a textured leather.

I love wearing different textures of the same color, and I've created many outfits using this beauty bundle. I've worn these same five pieces with a black lace skirt with subtle appliquéd flowers in the corner of it near the hem, and teamed it with a simple black silk sweater cut low in the back for dressier occasions. I've also loved this bundle with jeans and a crisp white shirt. I've worn

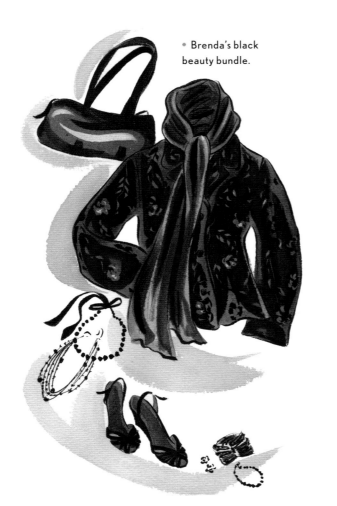

• Brenda's black beauty bundle.

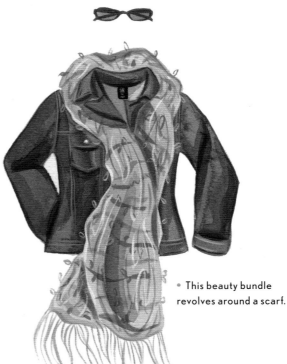

• This beauty bundle revolves around a scarf.

Thick loops woven into the scarf add interesting texture. It is truly a star piece—elegant, playful, and wild, all at the same time.

Since I was beginning with the scarf, I went to my closet to see what might relate to it. My jean jacket did. Great! And then I remembered these glasses with café lenses—not dark for wearing in pure sunlight, but tinted a shade of blue to wear in outdoor cafés with awnings. There was the start of a beauty bundle! I can dress for a casual date with friends in my key support piece, a pair of black pants; a T-shirt; and my jean jacket, which are all pretty basic. Then I throw that shawl over my shoulders or scrunch it up like a scarf and tie it in a big loose soft bow in front, add my blue

it with black pants and a black knit tank with sequins on it. With the same few pieces, I can go from dressy to casual. I'll change the shoes from pumps to sandals to boots depending on the time of year.

Now I'll demonstrate building a beauty bundle starting with an accessory, a scarf—well, a shawl really, but I wear it both ways. It's dramatic in a soft way. It's made of a sheer, gauzy wool netting in shades of dusty blue.

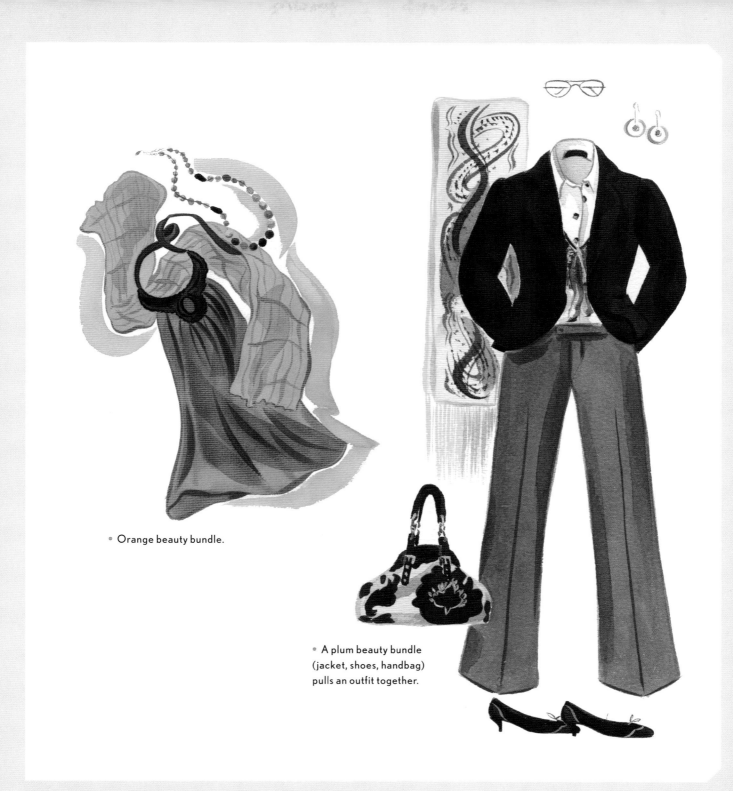

• Orange beauty bundle.

• A plum beauty bundle
(jacket, shoes, handbag)
pulls an outfit together.

café lenses, and simple dangly pearl earrings that go with anything. I stand out from everyone else in jeans and sweaters.

Can you see why I wanted you to group your accessories by color and see what you had? Accessories add interest and do a lot to make your outfit say more about you. They add layers to an outfit. Thinking about your things in beauty bundles will give you a jump start every time. If you find yourself rushing to get out of the house and you have one of your beauty bundles in mind, you hardly have to think.

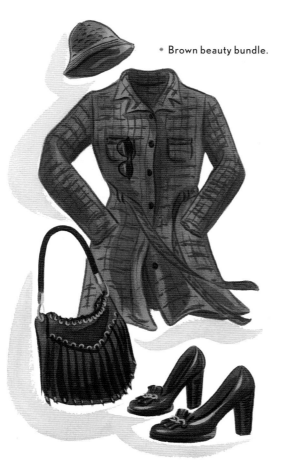

• Brown beauty bundle.

Write out your beauty bundles here. If they aren't complete, at least you know what you want to work on. Remember, a bundle has a minimum of three items.

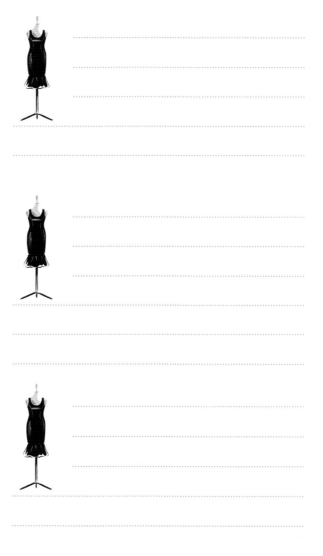

How did you do? Did you find a few diva-worthy bundles in your closet? Do you have some partial bundles? Decide what items are missing and put them on a shopping list. Then add whatever you need to complete each of the three outfits for your dates—dressy, casual, and at home. Underline any pieces that you need to bring with you if you're matching color, texture, or details. Don't take chances. Set yourself up for successful shopping by having a complete list and all the pieces that you need to work from with you. In the next chapter, I'll give you tips for successful shopping.

If you already have three complete outfits, write them down in your date plan on page 193. How about putting together some alternates? It's good practice. You should be able to describe each outfit with two or three of your style words.

Our next Diva Advisor has some tips on shopping vintage, which can be a perfect source of star pieces if you're in need of those. You might be inspired to take up vintage shopping for the fun of finding treasures. Diva Advisor Melissa Houtte is the coauthor of a book called *Alligators, Old Mink, and New Money,* which she wrote with her sister, Alison. (Alison, a former model, turned her love for fashion and vintage into a popular vintage shop in Brooklyn called Hooti Couture.) Melissa shares ideas for finding key star pieces for your wardrobe—and maybe your date outfits—from vintage stores. And the big advantage? You'll get lots of style without spending lots of money. You'll meet Alison on page 201.

• The star piece here is the bubble skirt. The scoop-neck sweater is the support piece.

THE VINTAGE ADVANTAGE

BY *Melissa Houtte*

✦

Add a handful of vintage pieces to your wardrobe, and see your look go from flavorless to fabulous. Vintage items are affordable, easy to find, and best of all, one of a kind. Look no further than your neighborhood vintage store or eBay. If you really like something, try it on. If it fits, grab it, because you may never see another one just like it. Here are my top ten vintage favorites:

1. Fifties cashmere cardigan. A gorgeous sweater, it works year-round with everything from jeans to a satin party skirt. Look for one with elaborate beaded trim or a rich fur collar (or one of each).

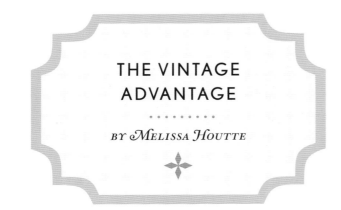

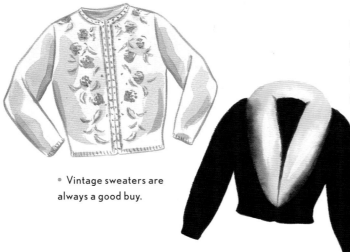

• Vintage sweaters are always a good buy.

2. An alligator or crocodile handbag from the '40s, '50s, or '60s. Many beautiful purses have no label, but if you want to be sure you get quality, you can't go wrong with Bellestone, Deitsch, or Lucille de Paris (look for their stamps inside). Do be careful when buying on eBay: some sellers label their bags as *'gator* or *crocodile* when, in fact, they are lizard or snake. Buy from sellers who have excellent feedback ratings and at least a hundred sales under their belts.

3. Velvet evening coat. With a red or black velvet evening coat from the '50s, '60s, or '70s, you are ready for anything.

4. Signed silk scarf. Wrap your neck in something soft and beautiful from Hermès, Pucci, Courrèges, Lanvin, or another famous designer. Or go with the more mainstream (and very affordable) Vera, whose strong colors and lively prints have aged well.

5. Pinup or pom-pom satin mules with a little heel. For your next dinner party, add a dash of glam! These delicious shoes can be flirty or just fun, and you can often find them unworn on eBay. The colors and styles vary; my favorite label is Daniel Green.

6. Vintage watch. If you are small-boned and petite, go for a woman's watch, preferably from the '40s, '50s, or '60s. Otherwise, try a man's watch for a bold, beautiful statement. I particularly love watches from the '40s in rose gold, with detailed faces and leather bands.

7. Cowboy boots. Boots add a sexy accent to jeans, and a good pair can last a lifetime, only getting better with age. But do look closely at the quality; you don't want anything that has begun to crack or flake. (The only time boots are a bad idea is in an airport security line. You won't look like much of a diva if you are struggling to pull the damn things off your feet while standing up.)

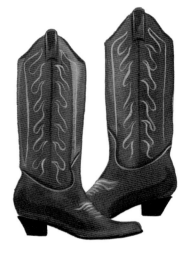

8. Wide rhinestone bracelet. Every diva wardrobe needs a certain amount of sparkle. If you want a piece that is collectible, look for one marked either *Weiss* or *Eisenberg*. But if you find a bracelet you like, and the clasp is good and strong, don't worry about who the maker is.

9. Silk nightgown, preferably from the '30s or '40s. At least a few nights each week, dump the T-shirts and flannel in favor of something that assures sweet dreams.

10. Faux leopard coat, '50s to '70s. Great coats abound in assorted styles, from trench to swing. Find the one that works for you, then wear it anytime you want to have fun.

BEAUTY SOAK This has been a very active few days. You really deserve this beauty soak! Get a cup of tea or coffee or other beverage of your choice, find your favorite sacred spot where you are at peace, whether it's on your porch, your chair in the front room, or in your bed, and do nothing. Absolutely nothing. Try to do nothing for twenty minutes. You'll feel recharged.

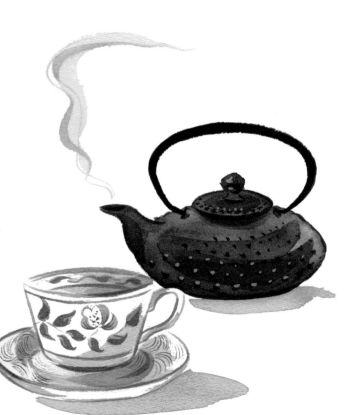

WEEK THREE

Chapter 11 • **SHOPPING**
PAGE 148

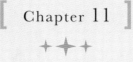

SHOPPING

No doubt you've discovered some holes in your wardrobe. I mean, no wonder it's been hard to dress your diva self, right? You've been missing some important star pieces, or your support pieces have lost their juice and need replacing and updating. You got started on a couple of beauty bundles that you're working into your date outfits. To complete your three outfits, maybe you need the right shoe or boot or sandal. Or do you need foundations?

You've been in your closet for days. Before I blow the shopping whistle, we have some ground rules to go over, some ruts to expose, and some things to think through. Stay with me now. There's so much to be distracted by. Everything's trying to get your attention—labels, brands, salespeople on commission, displays, price tags. It's a miracle people get anything right sometimes! But this time you're bringing a much sharper focus, which will make you a more powerful, effective shopper.

There are lots of shopping ruts that manage to sabotage people's efforts. Let's review some strategies to get out of those ruts:

1. Shop for what you love. "Kinda," "sorta," "close," or "it'll do" don't cut it anymore. This may be the first time you've gone shopping with the intention of fully satisfying yourself. You can do it!

2. Put yourself first. In the past you've spent money like it's water on kids, husband, nephews, and nieces. Well, diva, it's your turn!

3. Keep your eye on the prize. There's nothing more aging than looking dowdy, and dowdy is so not you anymore! By taking care of you, you'll be making everyone around you happier, too. Think of this as philanthropic work!

4. Looking your diva self is slimming, no matter what size you are. Remember to dress for the body you are currently in. You're spending money on what fits and flatters you now, not five months from now. You have dates to go on!

5. By shopping for the colors and styles you're clearly drawn to, you're honoring your diva style. Shop so you can show up.

6. Follow your plan and ignore everyone else's. If the fashion world is saying everyone needs a white shirt this season and it's not on your list, forget about it. You've worked out a plan. Stick to it.

7. Don't wait for the things you love to go on sale. You don't have time for that game now; you have dates to get dressed for. Remember the cost-per-wear formula. Divide the cost of something you want by the number of times you think you will wear it. That's your cost per wear. That $300 handbag, shoes, or jacket that you think you will wear constantly will be a bargain, even if you pay full price for it.

8. Don't give up. In Tai Chi class, my teacher reminds us that it takes a thousand repetitions to learn a series of movements, and then it becomes natural to us. But until then, we have to stay focused and concentrate. There's a lot of trial and error sometimes in shopping. Plus you're integrating a lot of new information about color, style, fit. Be willing to be a beginner, a student. You'll get good at this. You won't need a thousand repetitions, I promise.

9. Expect a good outcome. See it in your mind. Stop telling yourself the old stories about how you can't find things. You've got a new story to tell—how you found what you loved, it was easier than you expected, and you look great! That's your story. Stick to it.

IO. There are bonuses to finishing an outfit. Completing one whole outfit will do a lot for the rest of your wardrobe. The key things that have been missing could be the pieces that make another half dozen fabulous outfits complete. I see it all the time. When you solve one problem, there's a domino affect of unexpected benefits—including a lot of compliments.

Get out a piece of paper and make a new tic-tac-toe grid. You're going to use it to organize your shopping excursions. This time you're going to use all nine boxes. In the top row, from left to right, note at the top of each box the following three categories: "Star Pieces: Clothing, Underwear/Foundations, Shoes." In the second row, label the boxes "Belts/Bags/Scarves/Gloves/Sunglasses/Hosiery, Shopping Experience, Beauty Supplies." In the third row, from left to right, label the boxes "Jewelry, Outerwear, Support Pieces."

Stay focused on achieving success by shopping for exactly what you need right now for these dates. If you're working during this month, you may take a longer lunch hour, go to the beauty supply store, and check out the hair ornaments or products for your hair if those are in your Beauty Supplies box. You might tackle a shopping box one day after work. You'll make progress, step by step. Have you heard that saying "Inch by inch, it's a cinch. Yard by yard, it's hard"? I'm giving you the inch-by-inch plan because I want this to be a cinch for you. Every success builds upon the last one. Results will seem dramatic by the time you're only halfway through the list.

Give yourself rewards for each row that you complete, or if shopping is a major challenge for you, reward your efforts one box at a time! Start your rewards program here by writing in those things that would tickle your motivation. Dinner out? A trashy celebrity magazine and a bubble bath? Make it worth your effort if this is challenging. Rewards help!

STAR PIECES	UNDERWEAR/ FOUNDATIONS	SHOES
BELTS/ BAGS/ SCARVES/ GLOVES/ SUNGLASSES/ HOSIERY	SHOPPING EXPERIENCE	BEAUTY SUPPLIES
JEWELRY	OUTERWEAR	SUPPORT PIECES

Rewards Program

✦ ✦ ✦

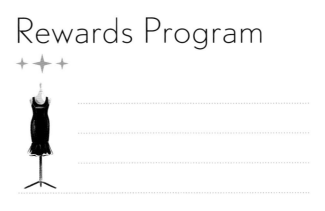

....

....

....

....

Next review any and all notes you've made about things you need to shop for. Start putting them in the grid under the appropriate category. You may have some categories that are empty, or they may all be full. The way these things are organized is the way you'll shop. You'll stay focused on one thing, complete it, and go to the next. Of course, I understand that you may accomplish several things in a day, but start out with the plan no matter what. It's a way of breaking up the tasks and keeping you on track. If you are shoe-challenged, take time to look at shoes and nothing else.

You can shop wherever you like. Some people like to shop where they can take things back with no hassles, such as department stores or chain stores. If you're more confident, you can shop at local boutiques, consignment stores, or design salons. Just be aware that they can't give you the return policy that a big chain store can if you're not happy. Don't be shy about asking for a twenty-four-hour approval period in which you can at least take it home and play with it for a while before you decide if it is right for you.

Keep to this basic rule wherever you shop: love it or find it useful. You don't have to totally be in love with your T-shirt bra, but you can appreciate its usefulness if it makes your body-conscious star piece look great.

If you're a die-hard bargain hunter, and shopping is your sport, please review the cost-per-wear formula before shopping anywhere. Just because it was cheap doesn't mean it was a bargain unless it really suits you. If you like to play games with money, here's a good one: The great deal you got on a blouse or the jacket you found at your local consignment store can be the bargain of the day. Now go out and buy the shoes with the price tag that's out of your normal comfort zone—only if they're right, of course. I never advocate buying designer anythings just because it has a designer's name attached to it. That will never get you diva status. How you put it all together will, and if all those pieces came from Goodwill, that's fine.

Save all of your receipts. If you are unsure about a purchase, staple the receipt to the hang tag while you decide. Then you won't be trying to find it when you have only twenty-four hours left before it's officially yours and not theirs.

DIVA SENSE

"I don't shop a lot, but I shop everywhere. If you're a good shopper, you can shop at T.J. Maxx and Loehmann's and find things that will work in your wardrobe. I'm open to things falling off the shelf at me. I have trust. I'll buy what I love and not worry if I don't have something to work with it. I know that within a couple of months, it will be part of a great outfit."

Cat

You've got the ground rules. And you have your list. So pull out your calendar and slot some shopping times for this week. Write them in your book as if they were appointments, because they are. Look at your calendar and estimate when you can get this shopping done. If you're shopping in malls, nighttime is great. Between five and nine in the evening, it's usually quieter. There are fewer customers, and salespeople are happy to spend time with you. Weekdays are less crowded than weekends. If there's a salesperson you like who makes things easier for you, find out her schedule and plan to see her then. If you want to try a personal shopping service in a store, call ahead and book time. It's important to give yourself the time and support you need to ensure success.

Okay, you've looked at your calendar. You've slotted some shopping times. I'm blowing the shopping whistle! Begin! Not sure where to start? Begin with whatever is most difficult for you. If, when you go shopping for bottoms, you always seem to come home with five tops instead, then start with bottoms. If you procrastinate when you need foundations and you haven't visited that department since, oh, let's say since high school, start there. Start with the thing you resist the most. I mean it! If you don't get a handle on it, you'll always believe that department has nothing for you, regardless of the store you're in. When you're shopping for the thing that's most difficult for you, don't keep it a secret. Tell the salesperson that you have a really hard time finding pants that fit you and ask for suggestions. Do the same thing in twelve stores; you may find solutions in unexpected places. It happens all the time. Believe me; you'll be trying on things you never considered because you're open to solutions. There are passionate salespeople out there who are geniuses about fit and product. I love it when I find these people! After working with them, you'll swear they were sent to earth just to solve pants problems. So be open. Trust that it's there. You are a dog after a bone; let your instincts lead you.

Working off your shopping grid, here are some tips for each section.

DIVA SENSE

"I take a lot of things into the dressing room at once so I can compare. I'll take in a pile of sweaters. When I try on the first sweater I may think, 'oh this is okay,' but as I try on more, I find others that are just so much better. I go back out and bring in another ten sweaters. If I had chosen just a few things, I might have bought the 'okay' sweater. The thing that's just okay doesn't seem like something to spend money on if you can eventually find something you love. It's not fun to buy things that give you a queasy feeling when you get home — those 'what was I thinking' pieces."

Karen

Star Pieces— Clothing

+ ✦ +

The star pieces of your outfits may end up being jewelry, handbags, or even shoes. If that is your goal, then adjust this section or just put stars next to the shopping areas where you expect to find your star pieces. Otherwise, think of this section as the one that will generate that fabulous off-the-shoulder top, a great jacket, stunning pants in a color or a pattern that only you could pull off, or a skirt that is so sexy and fun to wear.

Star pieces are the ones we naturally expect to pay more money for. Sometimes that's true, but not always. I've talked about a couple of star pieces of mine. Let me tell you how I shopped for them.

Last winter the Bellas —two friends and me— were getting together for a shopping excursion. The Bellas get together once a month. We used to meet to support each other in our businesses. Eventually we started supporting each other in our evolving styles, including all things fashion and beauty. I brought my images with me. I'd made a collage of things I loved and the direction I wanted to go in. When we arrived at one store, I immediately spotted a leopard print coat. It was the first thing I tried on. The Bellas were bubbling! "That's great on you!" they said.

It was from a vendor that I normally avoided and cost more than I wanted to spend but it made my heart go pitter-patter. I looked in the full-length mirror. I loved it yet it was a stretch for me. I opened up my wardrobe binder, and there was the assurance I needed: a picture of a leopard print coat similar to the one in the store. Wow! That's how resonance works! That's how doing your homework gets results. I never would have given that coat a second look. But there in my binder was a reminder of what I'd been drawn to. I'd never worn a print like that, but I was ready to get out of my comfort zone and try something new. I was a little nervous, but I bought it. I told myself I could always return it.

Within a few weeks—I had to wait for the weather to change—I pulled it out. It became my star piece. I wear it every which way, and I always get compliments. The colors are totally right for me, the fit is impeccable, and the fabric requires no special care. The cost-per-wear came down real fast.

I tell you this story because you might experience a similar situation—spending more and being a little nervous, or dressing in a way that makes you more noticeable and therefore uncomfortable. When we're not doing the same old thing we've always done, it can make us a little anxious. If you come across a piece that makes your heart pound, that could be a really good sign.

Diva Sense

"I bought this metallic jacket that was on the expensive side. But I know I can wear it after metallics have gone out of fashion because it's my hair color. It was made for me!"   *Karen*

When you're looking for star pieces, good places to check out are the departments in major department stores with the store's own labels. Generally you're getting a product that is a knockoff of a higher-end article that was a hit with a big-name designer, but for much less. You won't get the same fabric or details, but you'll have the same look. One of my favorite star pieces came from one of Macy's private lines. The look was very much like a Prada jacket that I loved, but a whole lot less expensive. It fit me perfectly. It was a black satin jacket patterned with a great jacquard floral design. The flowers seemed to go from light to dark because of the way they're woven into the fabric. It had beaded black buttons. Although it was on the floor with holiday clothes, I knew I could wear this anytime of the year. It appealed to that glamorous part of me that likes to look dressed up in casual clothes. I could wear it with velvet or satin pants or with jeans. This star piece is the best! Every time I wear it I get compliments. I keep the bargain part of it to myself, even though it's tough to do. I simply say, "Thank you."

When you're looking at star pieces, consider things that are in colors that really make a statement—a lime green sweater, a lilac silk blouse. If you choose a neutral color, like black, find something with interesting texture.

Underwear and Foundations

✦ ✦ ✦

I covered a lot about underwear and foundations in chapter 7. If you haven't gone on your underwear excursion, now's the time. I've had clients bring the outfit they planned to wear to a special event to the lingerie department. They were fitted for the proper foundations on the spot so we knew the outfit would look fantastic. I highly recommend this. Lingerie and foundation people are some of my favorites. They have so many solutions for us. They just need to be asked. With all the slimmers and shapers out there, there might be one that will make your outfit look better than ever. A well-fitting outfit makes you look wealthy and wise, so be smart and spend some time in this department. New products are being developed or improved upon all the time, so if you visited this department last year, you're still overdue for a checkup.

DIVA SENSE

"When I get new things, I want to enjoy them right away, even if I'm not wearing them yet. I'll take the item out of the bag, slip it onto a hanger, and hang it over my bedroom door so I can just keep looking at it. It's so beautiful and pleasing to me, I just want to enjoy it! It's like enjoying art. After a few days, I'll work it into an outfit, but I won't have missed a single bit of pleasure in the meantime." *Marj*

Shoes

✦ ✦ ✦

Many outfits are built around a shoe. What shoe is comfortable? What can you stand in for three hours? What can you walk in for three blocks? If you have a limousine service for your dressy date, this won't be an issue. Remember that when your feet aren't happy, you aren't either. You might love the high heels but if your feet don't, you might need to spend some extra time finding that shoe that will fit, flatter, and be functional all at once.

Always be on the lookout for shoes in metallic colors. They are perfect for blending outfits that have colorful patterns. If you try to match a color in a dress exactly, for example one with a pattern to it, you may look matronly. A metallic shoe becomes a neutral. If you wear silver jewelry a lot, find a shoe in pewter or a muted silver. It doesn't have to be shiny silver; just so it blends. The rule about shoes matching the hem of your skirt or pants is obsolete. Many people put color or pattern on the feet. Great idea. Try to bring the color up somewhere close to the face with an earring or necklace to tie it together. You also don't need to match shoes and handbags. That rule is gone too. However, I always find that if a shoe and a handbag blend, they can make many outfits work.

Don't try fitting into the same size shoe you wore ten years ago. Forget the size, and go for fit. And be open to ways to give your feet more comfort as well. Gel pads make the soles of your feet happier when you're in high heels.

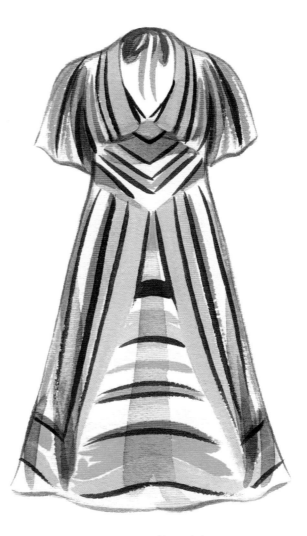

• Neutral shoes are great with prints.

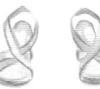

"I love good shoes for lots of reasons, but the prices pain my penny-pinching heart. So, here's what I do about it. I head for the 50-percent-off rack at my favorite high-end shoe store, knowing I will still spend a lot, somewhere between $100 and $200 a pair, and leave with shoes that I will wear for several years to come. I don't care if the shoes are already six months out of style because I don't focus on whether this minute's look is the kitten heel or the four-inch platform. I buy shoes that are distinctive, but not silly or gimmicky. They make my feet feel and look good and flatter my wardrobe. I know, from experience, that the quality of the leather and the design mean that these shoes will age much better than inexpensive shoes, even if I push them to the back of the closet for a year or two at a time, before returning them to action."

Melissa

Belts, Bags, Scarves, Gloves, Sunglasses, and Hosiery

✦ ✦ ✦

I've grouped these things together because they are generally treated this way in stores. This is probably my favorite department. Even in small boutiques, I'll walk in and check out these accessories before I look at the clothes. It's always the section I'll look at in the discount stores as well. If I'm hunting for belts, I can often find great ones for less than twenty dollars at those stores that sell lawn furniture and play equipment as well as clothes for the family. I've spent hundreds on a belt, too. I don't want you to think I'm not flexible!

Scarves and shawls are such wardrobe boosters. One everyday diva knitted a simple scarf for a special outfit she was wearing. She picked out a gold color in her printed long coat, found a luxurious yarn with a wonderful texture in a lighter shade, and got it done in time for her evening out. I can't even imagine the outfit without that scarf. It was a true diva detail.

One client finds art and function in gloves. She has a health condition that leaves her with cold hands and feet. No problem. She has gloves in many colors. They add unexpected accents to her clothes, creating great color combinations that actually turn leather gloves into a star piece.

Sunglass styles have their periods of being in vogue. Getting new ones can update your look.

Shopping Experience

✦ ✦ ✦

In the center of the tic-tac-toe grid it says "Shopping Experience." I want you to write a couple of words that will remind you of the type of experience you want. You might note the words *fun, affirming, relaxing,* or *adventurous*. Now think about how you will take care of yourself while you're shopping, and add that to the same box. Jot down your plan for taking breaks, bringing snacks or getting food, and possibly bringing a friend. Support yourself in new ways this time. Don't shop like you've shopped before. Create new and improved techniques for taking care of yourself.

Shopping can be challenging, but it can also be lots of fun, especially with reinforcements of food, water, and friendship. If you have a friend who's a great shopper (and is not bossy), ask her to join you.

Do you want to take a guess as to how many dresses Teri Hatcher, Felicity Huffman, or Susan Sarandon tries on before she settles on the one she wears down the red carpet? Do you think it might be 5? 10? 15? 25? Maybe 30? Could it possibly be 40? Try 50! A Hollywood stylist will arrange to have the movie star come to his or her loft, where fifty dresses have been assembled for her to try on. Food is set out and the space is made to be as comfortable and inviting as possible because it takes a long time to try on 50 dresses. And then the dress has to be fitted to the actress.

Treat yourself like a queen. Shopping is a real leveling field. It can try the patience of the most skilled surgeon, the toughest litigator, the fiercest mom, the most tenacious city reporter. Make it fun! Plan for success before you even get into your car. Gather your shopping list, your plan, and any items that you want to bring in order to complete your outfits. Pack your snacks and put on your walking shoes.

Beauty Supplies
✦ ✦ ✦

If you decided to start early on your hair, makeup, and skin care updates, you probably have a list of items to shop for. If you don't have a list, you will soon enough! There may be things you already know you want, like hair ornaments, a set of hot rollers, or a magnifying makeup mirror. Put those items in this box now. After you've spent more time with your hair and makeup, plan to come back here and fill in with the items you'll need to get ready for your dates. When you're shopping favorite lines of makeup or skin care, give yourself time to ask the questions, get the sample products, try on some of the things you're considering. Also, consider searching out the best hair dryer, makeup brushes, and any other tools you'll need to execute your look. Do this first if you never seem to get around to buying these. Getting your beauty products and tools together will assist you greatly in putting the look together. This could be a miniproject in itself, so please allow enough time.

Jewelry
✦ ✦ ✦

You should never opt out of finishing an outfit because you think the accessories will break the bank. I was in a shoe store where the starting price was around six hundred dollars. The salesperson in this chic shoe boutique looked fabulous. I complimented her on her necklace, and she immediately confessed the source — Target. "I'm not going to pay a lot for jewelry trends that may be gone quickly," she explained. Now this is something I don't want you to do — ever! Go ahead and shop the discount places for fashion pieces if you like, but never confess your sources! If you're looking fabulous and someone compliments you, just say "Thank you." They don't have to know whether that necklace is $12.95 or $1,295.

Another source for accessory pieces is the junior department of major stores. Don't even think about trying to get into the T-shirts, but do look at the jewelry. That's where you'll find instant style for a lot less money than the things in the finer costume jewelry departments in another part of the store. Or shop local craft shops or larger farmers' markets.

You might be shopping for a pricier signature piece. This could be a necklace that takes your breath away and says "you" for the next thirty years. Although I'd look silly in traditional dainty pearls, when I came across a classic double-stranded pearl necklace in bronze, I resisted for a few days, but couldn't get them out of my head. I splurged. The first time I wore them was to a monthly meeting of a group of friends. I put them with a simple caramel-colored T-shirt, a pearlized blond leather jacket, and a pair of jeans. The compliments came pouring in. There are days when I wake up in the morning and start constructing my outfit based on those pearls. They work with my coloring, and are classic but unexpected because of their color, which appeals enormously to my sensibilities. Plus they're fabulous year-round. That's a signature piece! By the way, I bought these pearls in a designer's private salon. Independent jewelry designers often have their own shops and are good places to check out.

When shopping for a signature piece, be patient. Let it draw you in, get under your skin, and into your mind. A signature piece is one you stick with over time. A trendy piece doesn't need to meet that criteria. It can be a temporary, inexpensive addition to your jewelry collection.

Be sure to finish a jewelry story that you start. If you fall for a necklace or bracelets, be sure you have earrings that will work with them. Remember, they don't have to match, just relate in some way. If you pick up some brooches, repeat something about the brooch in the earrings. If the brooch has crystals, diamonds, or a metal color, such as gold, wear crystal, diamond, or gold earrings.

DIVA SENSE

"If I find a basic top that works, I buy it in two of every color that flatters me. That way if one is in the laundry or at the cleaners, I still have a top to wear." *Karen*

DIVA SENSE

"I've been building up my good jewelry collection with the money that I'd spend on a boyfriend if I had one. I just decided that until I get that boyfriend who will buy me those things, I'm going to buy myself something special each year, wrap it up, and put it under the tree. Other people get those special big holiday gifts. Why not me? My 'boyfriend' has given me diamond hoops, a diamond ring, amethyst earrings, and this year he's giving me a diamond bracelet. In a weird way it makes me feel independent that I'm buying myself these things. I can do it myself. I don't need someone else to buy it for me." *Amy*

Outerwear

✦ ✦ ✦

There's nothing worse than putting together a great outfit and then heading to the coat closet, only to discover that none of your coats will work with it. You hope to just slither into your function unnoticed. Well, no diva does that and gets away with it. She shouldn't even attempt it! Get your outerwear in order. Coats that you won't wear often are great things to look for in consignment stores, outlet stores, discount stores, and vintage shops. Also check the sale racks in better department stores. A salesperson once told me that no one should ever pay full price for a coat. Once a season is over, stores are anxious to dump their inventory, and that's a good time to get a stash of proper outerwear. Usually if your outfit contains the star piece, your coat needs to be more neutral, devoid of attention-getting devices like huge pockets or lots of hardware.

Capes and shawls are great alternatives to coats because they're softer and less tailored than a coat and work well with formal and informal clothing. On the other hand, finding a coat in a bright color, metallic color, or in satin is a great way to turn this functional item into a star piece. I have a black chenille coat with faux zebra trim on it. I don't wear it often, but it's perfect for special occasions. Oh, and in case you missed your hall closet when you were cleaning out your closet, do it! Usually three-quarters of what's in a hall closet is dated and will make you look likewise.

● Dramatic outerwear adds fun to your outfit.

● Hem pants on the long side to give you long legs.

Support Pieces

+ + +

The trick with support pieces is to stay on top of them. The day our favorite pair of pants turns on us and comes out of the dryer two inches shorter is the day we go out and buy a new pair of pants. Same with tops, underwear, and some classic shaped sweaters. If a moth attacked your one cashmere sweater tomorrow, what would you be wearing if you depended on it? Some things need regular replacing—black and white T-shirts or whatever colors you rely on the most for instance. Keep the list of your support pieces in your wallet, including style numbers. You'll be so happy you took care of yourself this way!

Diva Does Alterations

+ + +

Handle your alterations right away. Hem things on the long side if they're supposed to be long. Ask the tailor to show you how it would look with a break in the pants. More fabric is more luxurious, more expensive-looking, more diva! Don't skimp. Even if you're budgeting and being careful, it doesn't have to show. Remember how dorky guys looked when they wore high-water pants? It puts the dowdy into the diva. Same with sleeve lengths. A quarter of an inch longer than standard will make you look more fashion forward, more on top of it, more diva.

Once you've completed your shopping, bring your things home and try them on. Put together your beauty bundles. Add the star pieces and the support pieces. Do you have the shoes and handbag that you need? How does everything look? Are the outfits complete? Do they express your style? Maybe you're close but you want to have another little mini–closet session and try a few other combinations. An outfit you started working on might be less interesting to you now that you finished a beauty bundle. You may have discovered something else in your closet that you like even better. That's allowed! You can change your mind! Keep working toward those three fabulous date outfits.

With the tags still on the pieces you've purchased, test drive each outfit by walking around the house and seeing how it feels, sitting down and seeing how the fabric responds to creasing, standing back up and viewing yourself in a full-length mirror from all angles.

If some things are not right, pack them up, return them, and start again, fine-tuning your shopping list based on how this first one went. Expect to do some returning and some more shopping. You're learning lots of things along the way, and hopefully they will make shopping easier for you in the long run. You have your vision for how you want to look for your dates. Stick to it. You have a whole week to work on this. The rewards will be worth it! Have fun!

Your dates will be here sooner than you realize. You're going to want photographs taken to mark the special occasions. Whether they're taken by your partner, daughter, or a hired professional, you want to look terrific in them. Our Diva Advisor Bernie Burson knows just how to pose for a photo so you will be happy with it. All those bad photos in the past? Not your fault. Bernie has worked alongside an advertising photographer and has a keen interest in looking decent in pictures. Check out her tips. And then see if you can get some practice in before those dates arrive so you remember just where to put your hands and just how much to tilt your head. Smile!

Coming up next are your hair and makeup appointments. Look how far you've come! These first weeks have been the most intense. You've done a lot of work to get to this spot. Your upcoming hair and beauty treatments will be just the pampering you deserve. And of course, another beauty soak is in order! Then we'll be back in your closet getting ready for your dates. See you soon!

BEAUTY SOAK Since you're out shopping this week, let's make your beauty soak a shopping experience as well. Take a break from clothes shopping and change your focus. Do you have something you love to buy? Greeting cards? Nail polish? Books? CDs? Magazines? Keep the sticker price low, take a breather from your outfits, and indulge yourself in one of your favorite things to shop for. You need a break from all this concentration. Enjoy!

HOW TO HAVE YOUR PICTURE TAKEN

BY BERNIE BURSON

Many of us hate the way we look in pictures and assume we're just not photogenic. While it's true that the camera loves some bone structures more than others, it is possible to improve your chances of looking good in photos.

First, you need to understand that the camera sees things in only two dimensions, height and width. It doesn't allow for depth. In other words, what is closer looks larger, and what is farther away looks smaller. You can position yourself strategically to take advantage of this phenomenon.

Let's start with your face. Most people unconsciously tip their heads back slightly as they smile. This causes the cheeks (where most of us are wider) to be closer to the camera, and the eyes to be farther away. The resulting photograph shows a big smile, chubby cheeks, and squinchy eyes.

The way to avoid this is to tip your head slightly forward as you smile. This puts more emphasis on your eyes and less on your cheeks, giving your face a slimmer, wider-eyed appearance. The trick here is to keep the forward tilt *slight* — otherwise, you'll look like you're trying to be sultry. Here's an easy way to determine the right amount of tilt: Hold your head straight, put your index finger horizontally under your nose, and slide it down to the top of your lip. Now hold your finger still and bring your nose down until it hits your finger. It's only about half an inch, but it makes a big difference.

For full-length pictures, stand with one foot forward and perpendicular to the other; weight is on the back foot. Your body should be at an angle to the camera. This creates a slimmer, more elegant effect than a straight-on stance. Leave your hands relaxed at your sides. If you clasp your hands in front of you, your tummy will be emphasized.

For seated photos, turn your knees a bit to one side and have one foot slightly in front of the other. Only those with the slimmest thighs should consider crossing their legs. Sit up straight and lean forward just a little.

Never let anyone take your picture from below. The angle is terribly unflattering, and you will look haughty or downright mean.

Don't try to widen your eyes when you smile — let them crinkle naturally. Wide eyes are okay with a small or lips-only smile. With a big smile, wide eyes look demented.

Don't stand with a frozen smile while the photographer fiddles with the camera. Ask for a "ready" signal, then look toward the camera and smile naturally. If you think your smile looks too "grinny," press your tongue against your front teeth, then smile.

It should make you feel better to know that not even models look great in every photo. Professional photographers often take several rolls of film to get the perfect shot.

Finally, when choosing among several photographs of yourself, hold them up to a mirror. This is how you're accustomed to seeing yourself, and part of the reason you think your pictures don't look quite right.

There now! Ready for your close-up?

WEEK FOUR

Chapter 12 • **HAIR**

PAGE 166

Chapter 13 • **MAKEUP**

PAGE 176

Chapter 14 • **DIVA DATES**

PAGE 189

Chapter 15 • **DIVA FOREVER**

PAGE 203

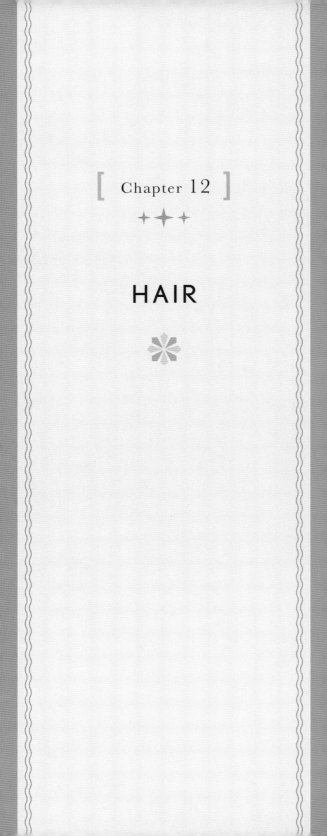

[Chapter 12]

✦ ✦ ✦

HAIR

❋

The first two weeks you stayed at home and worked on getting your CSF (color, style, fit) formula. You put beauty bundles together, and figured out what you needed to shop for to complete your three outfits. Last week you took care of the shopping. Now, in Week Four, you'll head off to your beauty appointments and finish getting ready for your dates. Then you're off to have fun in your new diva style!

DIVA SENSE

"Getting ready to go to your high school reunion can be really stressful. I was glad to have found an outfit in my closet that was really me: a patterned sleeveless dress, shrug sweater, and interesting and expressive jewelry. But I knew that the outfit wasn't going to work without great hair. I did the smart thing and I got a professional blow-dry. I was so comfortable at the reunion. I had the most fun ever!"

Lynn

If you're like most women, your hair is a sore subject—it's too thick, too thin, too curly, or too straight. Wouldn't it be interesting if your hair became your best asset? I've got a story to tell about that! It's also important to give some thought to what you're going to do with your hair for your special dates. You could try something new. I'm going to lay out lots of options—a professional blow-dry, a fresh new color or a fresh new cut, hair accessories, and more. This is the week to step it up a notch when it comes to your hair.

If you've neglected your hair or gotten confused about how to deal with it, you may be in a serious rut. In this chapter, I'm going to guide you out of your rut and set you up for gorgeous, luxurious hair success. I'll do what I can to give you good tips, but it's essential that you find a good stylist to work with. Hair stylists are full of information, and all you have to do is ask. In this chapter, Diva Advisor Dawn Litton, a stylist and instructor, will help you develop a fabulous relationship with a stylist—your partner in beauty. Whether you're looking for someone new or just want to get more talent out of the stylist you already have, Dawn's tips will help you get the most out of your hair appointment.

Let me tell you about Peggy. I met her during a makeover project for a magazine in Stockholm. All her life her hair had brought her only misery. She had naturally curly hair, which she tried to beat into submission every day with a hair dryer and a round brush, pulling, tugging, and trying to get it straight and smooth. She was working against her hair, not with it! Little did she know that her hair was really one of her best assets—adorable, curly hair. We gave her a great cut and showed her how to use some products. Suddenly, her hair became one of her most flattering features. The curls framed her face and brought attention to her pretty eyes and lips, something her straight hair couldn't do. She looked like a movie star. Best of all, now that she didn't have to spend an hour each day with the blow-dryer, she had more time to spend with her family in the mornings. Years of frustration vanished.

Many of us are guilty of working against our hair. You know who you are. Recently I came across this sign outside a hair salon in my town: "Life is an endless struggle filled with frustration and challenges . . . but eventually you find a hairstyle you like." I might consider adding this line: "Or, you finally accept the hair you have and make the most of it."

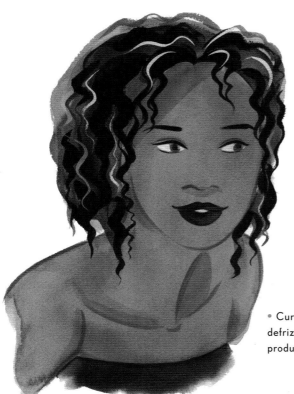

• Curly hair is tamed with defrizzers and other styling products.

Hair Ruts

✦ ✦ ✦

"Women over forty should wear short hair." How many times have we heard that? Is it true? No, you can wear your hair short, long, any length you want. Change is good! Difficult sometimes, but good! Let's talk about some hair ruts that could be standing in the way of your diva style.

1. Tight perms. You know the look: A cap of tight curls, often with very dry, unhealthy ends. Perms have evolved. Your hair doesn't have to be kinky in order to have body and a bend to the hair. If you've been in a perm rut, be willing to have a serious listening session with your stylist as she or he explains options.

2. Frosting. Frosting is for cakes, not hair. Making hair ends look white was a popular trend decades ago. Highlights or lowlights will add dimension to hair and make you look much younger and healthier. Frosting is a very dated look. If you got stuck there, time to get unstuck.

3. Long hair with straight bangs. Longer hair with straight bangs is a younger hairstyle. It looks terrific on twelve-year-olds, but on older women, it's aging. Long hair without bangs can be beautiful, though, especially if it's healthy, well groomed, and the ends are trimmed regularly so they don't split.

4.   Puffy '80s bangs. A much more flattering look is a side part with a tapered bang that grazes the forehead as it goes from shorter to longer.

5.   Wash-and-wear hair. Wash-and-wear hair is a myth. There are cuts that don't require a lot of work, but everyone should put some effort into styling their hair each day — even if just reviving yesterday's blowout.

6.   Dyed hair that's too dark. Nature intended to do us a favor by graying our hair, adding softness to our faces as they gain lines on them. Hair dyed too dark makes the lines of the face appear deeper. Better to go a shade or two lighter than a shade or two darker.

7.   Shapeless gray hair. Gray hair can be absolutely stunning if styled in a fresh, modern cut. Leaving it long and shapeless will really bring you down. It's not going to do anything for your diva style.

8.   Teasing through the top. Think of the TV show *Dynasty* with Joan Collins. This look is twenty years old. Weight distribution is crucial to a modern look. If you used to wear your hair with a lot of volume at the top and in the front, you need to stop. It's better to have volume through the crown area; it creates a nice profile. Retro hairstyles come back in vogue, but be careful doing this the second time around.

9.   Pigtails. One of the most surreal interviews I saw on TV was actress and ThighMaster mogul Suzanne Somers sitting on a couch talking about the merits of being over fifty. She was wearing her hair in braided pigtails, a look that better suits preadolescent girls. It was impossible to take her seriously. Hair pulled back into a ponytail can be sleek on some women, but not pigtails.

10. Center parts. It's a rare occasion when a center part flatters anyone over the age of twenty. An uneven part can be an attractive alternative.

DIVA SENSE

As a hairstylist, it would just kill me every time Judy came in wanting a perm. She was stuck in the '80s. Finally I said, 'Let me do your hair the way I think it would be good on you. Watch how I style it. I'll send you home with the products I use, and you try it at home. Then promise me you'll give me one more chance. If you don't like it after the second cut, we'll go back to the perm.' I wanted a chance for her friends to tell her how great she looked. It worked. I had her grow out her perm and it took ten years off of her. She came back and said, 'All my friends are telling me how great I look.' It was a more natural look on her and was easy, too."   *Thyra*

Finding a Hairstylist

✦ ✦ ✦

Hairstylists really want what's best for you. If you look good, they look good. They have a lot to teach you about your hair if you let them. To find a good one, look around you. Whose haircuts do you admire? Ask for referrals from friends. Someone in your office, car pool, or book group may have some great recommendations, too. The best stylists I've found have all come from referrals. Go in for a consultation. Most stylists offer free consultations. Keep looking until you find a good fit. And remember, getting your hair done should be a pampering, nurturing experience. So if you're with someone who is not pleasant, move on. You should really enjoy this beauty time. Also keep in mind that it's not necessary to stick with just one person for all aspects of your hair. I know that our loyalty to hairdressers is sometimes stronger than our loyalty to our husbands. You might want a colorist and a stylist. In fact, one salon owner I spoke with suggested using several people within a salon. That way if you your hair needs attention and the person who usually styles your hair is unavailable, you've got backup.

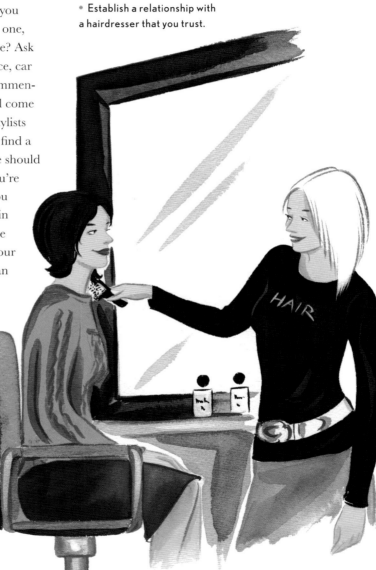

• Establish a relationship with a hairdresser that you trust.

HOW TO WORK WITH YOUR HAIRDRESSER

· · · · · · · · · ·

BY DAWN LITTON

✦

1. Shop around for a hairstylist. Find someone who's a good fit and seems to understand your concerns. When you're comfortable with someone, you may be more willing to try something new. Do a consultation with a few different people so you find someone you can let go with. Some women want their hand held, others need someone who will be firm with them. It's best to know who you are. Once you've found the right person, trust her or him. It's so much fun when my clients trust me. I feel that's when they get the best work out of me. They can relax in the chair, so it's a better experience all around.

2. Be open with your hairdresser. I put my energy into clients who are flexible and look to me for advice. If someone is rigid or snotty, I won't bother. The more open people are, the more willing I am to give.

3. Bring in pictures of what you like and don't like. Both are useful.

4. Tell your hairdresser anything that could possibly be useful to her. Most bad haircutting experiences are a result of bad communication.

5. Tell your hairdresser what kind of statement you want to make with your hair. Do you want to look arty? Sophisticated? Sexy? You can use hair to express your personality.

6. Don't be afraid to open up to your stylist about medical or personal issues that may affect your hair: thyroid, menopause, going through chemo, emotional issues like going through a divorce. You could be dealing with a new hair texture if you're dealing with health issues and medications.

7. Don't wear your hair too light or too dark. You may have been blond at the age of five, but that doesn't mean light blond flatters you now. Hair that's too dark looks inky and dense. It's hard looking. Natural tones are always better. Avoid eggplant or maroon. If you want to look funky, do it with your haircut.

8. Use your product! So many people buy tons and tons of products and never use them. I want my clients to use them so they look cute every day. It's the only way to duplicate what we do in the salon.

9. If you tell your hairdresser "Do whatever you think best," you had better mean it!

Scalp and Hair Care for Women over Forty

✦ ✦ ✦

Finding someone who can style and color your hair is one thing, but what you do with your hair in between appointments is up to you. Healthy hair needs your help. Here are my tips for hair care:

1. Avoid washing your hair every day. As your body ages, it produces less oil. You strip the hair of essential oils when you wash it too frequently. Your hairdresser can help you choose a shampoo that will protect your hair.

2. Take care of your scalp by giving it weekly scalp treatments or by brushing your hair every day with a boar bristle brush. Those one hundred strokes with a boar brush, done with a rolling motion with your wrist, can stimulate the scalp and spread the oils throughout your head of hair. It only takes about three minutes, and it's one of those things that can help your mental well-being simply because you're doing something good for yourself. As a bonus, it's sort of meditative.

3. Don't get obsessive about cleaning a boar bristle brush. It only has the oils from your hair in it and that's good. Just pull the hair from it and clean it that way.

4. If you're losing hair, don't be afraid to brush it. I know it sounds counterintuitive, but that hair died a month ago. You're not disrupting anything by continuing to give your hair good care.

5. Invest in shampoo and conditioner that are right for your hair texture and any coloring you've had done to your hair. Your stylist should be advising you on how to preserve and protect your investment. A lot of shampoos are really strong and work fine on regular hair, but they can strip the color right off.

Diva Sense

"I went to a new hairdresser when I felt my old one had done all he could for me. He seemed to be stuck in a rut. This new person was really young. She stood behind me, pushed at my hair, pulled at it, and finally said authoritatively, 'Long. We need to grow it long.' I was over fifty and had worn my hair short my whole life. No one had ever said that to me. I was stumped. I argued. She said, 'No, when it's long it will be sexy, inviting, luscious.' Those words resonated with me. I grew my hair out over the next year or two, and she was right. It was all those things. I never had so much fun."

Connie

Going Gray

✦ ✦ ✦

I am often asked about what colors to wear with gray hair. Some gray hair has warmer tones, and some gray hair has cooler ones. The women who talk about their gray hair in the following Diva Senses share the same hair color but nothing else. Debra S. has golden skin tones, moss-green eyes, and gray hair in a mixture of warm and cool shades. The last time we met, she was wearing a brown ribbed turtleneck, a camel-colored embroidered brushed corduroy jacket, a long jean skirt, and brown wedged shoes. She carried a red handbag. She was an everyday diva! And she was breaking a commonly held belief that warm tones aren't great with gray hair. She looked great in these warm colors because she has warmth in her coloring. Kathy has very silvery gray hair and has always worn cool colors best, even before she turned gray. Now she wears mostly bright white, black, and metallic shimmery gray colors. She could never wear the colors Debra S. does. So if your hair is graying and you're keeping it that way, you will most likely make adjustments in your color palette, but not necessarily in the color temperature of your palette.

You might want to adjust your makeup and accessories if you keep your gray hair. It's important to add some luster or light to your face, and you can do that with makeup that has some sheen in it, rather than matte. Or wear necklaces or earrings that bring light to your face—diamonds, crystals, and semiprecious and precious stones.

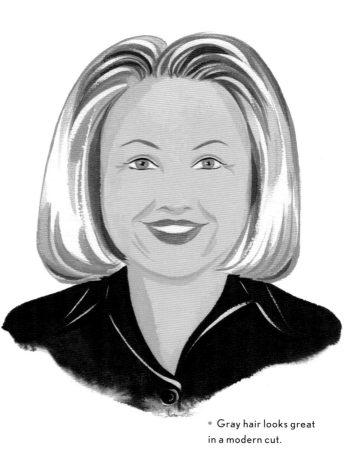

• Gray hair looks great in a modern cut.

Upkeep

✦ ✦ ✦

You'll need regular haircuts. The frequency depends on the complexity or the length of your cut. Shorter hair usually needs to be trimmed more often than longer hair. If time and money are an issue, ask your hairdresser for a cut that isn't too high-maintenance.

Then you'll need to learn how to style your hair at home. You'll want to know what tools you need and which products to use. Good products can enhance your hair by helping with volume, control, texture, shine, and hold. You won't be able to create the same shapes or looks as the hairdresser does without product such as straightening gel, defrizzers, curl cream, wax, volume sprays, and even hair mascara. Every time you change your hairstyle, talk to your stylist about hair products.

Every style will require different products. Bring your products from home, the ones that tumble out of the lower bathroom cabinet when you go looking for something, and ask your hairdresser if they are still relevant to your hair cut and texture at the moment. Toss the ones that aren't appropriate for your hair anymore, or give them to a homeless shelter.

Styling techniques can be learned. Sure, there's nothing like a styling from a professional, and you might choose this option for your dates. Having someone else style your hair will certainly make it less stressful for you, and the styling can often last you a week. But between haircuts you may want to book half an hour of the stylist's time and let her teach you how to do some simple things at home. Or bring in hair ornaments and let her show you some quick ways to put your hair up or back to make it look special. She may show you how to add glosses for shine or other products that are good for your particular style. Your stylist is an incredible resource for you, and it's wise to learn as much as you can so you're able to give your hair the special treatment it deserves.

You've had a lot of years with your head of hair, but someone taking a fresh look at it could give you a whole new perspective on life. Don't be stubborn or uncooperative. See if you can trust someone to do a good job. Go into your appointment looking your best diva self, with makeup on, great shoes, jewelry, the works. Show the person who you are. It will help her or him understand how best to serve you.

Once you've built a relationship with a stylist you like, learn to book your appointments far enough ahead to secure the dates you need, especially during the holidays or when you're going on a trip. If there are special occasions coming up (like your three dates!), you might want to schedule that blow-dry. If you end up with someone other than your regular stylist, that could be a good thing, too. Remember, they all went to school to get there. You're most likely in good hands.

A good haircut and coloring brings your face into focus. Your hair is art for your face. Take care of that artwork. Go back for extra lessons for using product and styling your hair. If you're suffering from hair loss, get a referral from your hairdresser for someone who can help. You may decide to go with a wig or a hair piece that will fill in your hair. Don't stay home and be miserable. You've got dates to go on! Find the solutions. Book those appointments. Promise?

BEAUTY SOAK When I go to get my hair done, it is a supreme beauty soak experience. What's not to love about someone running their fingers through my hair and giving me neck massages? You may feel that way too. If you're going to your hair appointments this week, you might count that as your beauty soak activity. But I bet you could still fit in time for a movie. How about curling up and watching a couple of great hair movies? Both of them revolve around hairdressers who want to open their own shop. *Shampoo*, the 1975 classic comedy, stars Warren Beatty, Goldie Hawn, and Julie Christie. *Beauty Shop*, a 2005 comedy, stars Queen Latifah, Kevin Bacon, and Andie MacDowell. Also check out how well Queen Latifah puts outfits together. I recommend watching these as a double feature!

Diva Sense

"When I walk out to the street after seeing my hairstylist, all fatigue from the day is gone. I feel like running into my ex-boyfriend or going to a hotel bar and ordering an apple martini, even though my perfect mate has dinner waiting for me at home. I feel lifted from ordinary life. I could play hooky and not call the kids, not call my parents, head for the airport, and board a plane for anywhere. That's what a good cut and color does for me. It spins my world around, lightens my load, shaves five years and ten pounds off my driver's license stats. I do go home for dinner, but I bring all that excitement with me."

Bridget

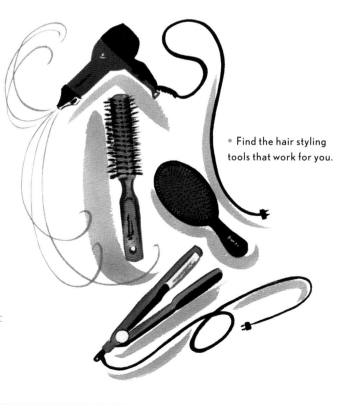

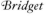 Find the hair styling tools that work for you.

[Chapter 13]

✦ ✦ ✦

MAKEUP

✳

If you've been sailing along thinking you've handled all your ruts, you've just come to a chapter that could make you stumble. Lots of women get stuck in makeup ruts, and we'll take care of those this week. Every diva needs a makeup update. If you haven't had one in a while, you'll get some good tips here. Makeup works best on healthy skin, and you'll learn about skin care as well.

Although you may have done a great job of getting your outfits together, makeup and grooming is necessary to give you polish. The right makeup makes you look fresher, more vital. Good makeup products and techniques and a solid skin care regimen may be all you need to move into the next decade feeling great about yourself. I'm not going to be talking about face-lifts or other procedures that would require a visit to a doctor's office. That's more research and recovery time than you've got in order to be ready for your diva dates! But if this is something that's on your mind, start putting your feelers out for some good referrals. In Diva Forever, the last chapter, you can transform those ideas into plans for the future.

Changes

✦ ✦ ✦

As we get older, our hair, eyes, and skin can get lighter. We might lose eyebrows. The texture of our skin is different. The way we take care of our skin and use makeup products needs to change to meet our new needs.

Makeup—the eye shadows, the concealers, high-lighters, and lipsticks you use—help us see you more clearly. The right products applied with the proper techniques will add definition to your features. I don't want you ever to suffer from invisibility! Aging doesn't mean disappearing. No way. When your features are in focus, we can see your beauty and vitality. That's where we're headed.

If you've been away from makeup and skin care products for years, you'll find that formulations and

techniques have changed. It's an industry that evolves. Chances are much of what's in your makeup stash expired years ago, and for good reason. Better things have replaced them, which means there are better solutions out there for you. I want to help you find them. In addition, two Diva Advisors will be with you in this chapter. Felicia will address your skin care regimen. And Lynn is going to help you find a lipstick that's just right for you.

Maybe you've been addicted to Bubblegum Pink lipstick. And even when it was discontinued fifteen years ago, you kept carrying around that last tube

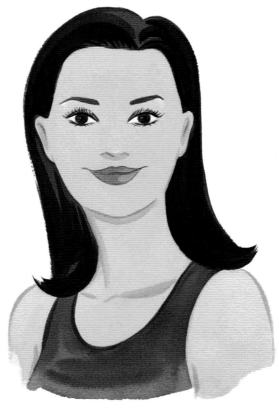

• Go for a healthy, not overly made-up look.

trying to replace it with the next closest thing. Your Bubblegum Pink obsession is blinding you from new products that would be so much more appropriate and better looking on you. It's time to let go of the past.

If you have taken care of your skin diligently, you're still looking at a different face in the mirror from the one you saw decades ago. Gravity is changing the contours of your face. Your eyes are receding. Their color may be softening. It's hard to know how to dress up this face. Let's talk about some common mistakes and work toward the solutions.

Common Mistakes
✦ ✦ ✦

1. Visible concealer. Concealer products should be only a tiny bit lighter than your skin tone. You shouldn't be getting those white raccoon lines under your eyes. Your skin tone may have changed, so getting this color right is important.

2. The wrong foundation color. It's tough to get this right, especially if you're pulling colors off a rack in a drugstore. Even someone at a makeup counter may steer you in the wrong direction. If you're experimenting with a few shades, test them on your jaw line, not your hand. The one that's right should really disappear into your skin. As we age, our face gets texture—wrinkles, crow's feet, larger pores. It's important to adjust your foundation to this change in texture. If you have age spots and you find the foundation that's right for you, it will make them seem to disappear and give you an overall natural look, as if you have no makeup on at all.

3. Unruly eyebrows. As we age, the eyebrows become more sparse. They don't keep a shape. Try getting your eyebrows shaped by a professional. You'll find you may look as if you had an eye lift. Our eyesight isn't as good, and it's hard to do this for ourselves, so we ignore it. If you aren't good at this, it is worth working this service into your beauty regimen every four to six weeks. You can have it done at the same time as your facial or see a professional makeup artist.

If you want to shape your brows at home yourself, fill them in as you would normally with a pencil or powder. Then tweeze. This way you won't be likely to pull out some hairs that appear to be stragglers but actually are in the line of where your eyebrows should be. There are stencils that you can buy to help. There's almost nothing that is more important to giving definition to your face than shaping your brows.

4. Botched blush. Too much blush makes you look like a clown. It's best to use less blush than you did years ago, and back off of bright colors on the cheeks. You might need a different type of blush as well. As we age, we lose some of the natural dewiness in our skin, cream blushes can be so much easier to use than powders.

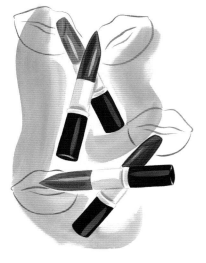

• Lipsticks need updating every year.

5. Updates that aren't. When you stopped by the makeup counter in a department store and picked up a new eye shadow color, you didn't get an update, you got a new product. When you get an update, you consult with a makeup artist who evaluates your current regimen with you, studies your face, reviews the current trends in makeup, and shows you products and techniques that are right for you. Schedule one while you're going through beauty camp. I'll give you ideas about how later. You may need to teach your fingers new tricks. Most people continue to apply their makeup exactly as they have for years. Their fingers go to the same spots, and apply the same pressure out of habit. A lighter touch may give you better results now. Again, a professional can best give you a new plan and train your hand how to do it.

6. Color coding to your outfit. Trained professionals might be able to pull this off, but as we mature, it's really not necessary. If your eyelids are puffy or crepey, that's not where you want to be wearing lime green. You don't need to match your clothes to your makeup in order to look pulled together.

7. Relying on makeup counters for all your advice. A twenty-two-year-old may not understand your needs the way someone would who is closer to your age.

8. Seeing lines. Lining the lips and filling in with a lighter color so the liner still shows is not good. Neither is wearing an eyeliner that is too thick and heavy. Seeing a foundation line is not good. Everything should be blended, blended, blended.

9. Falling victim to the latest "in" color. We don't need to change our makeup regimen every six months. It's true that makeup has seasons and trends just like clothes do. But a look that is consistent and somewhat flexible—giving you the option of changing your lipstick or eyeliner for example—is more realistic.

Skin Care

+ ✦ +

So where do you start? Good makeup starts with good skin care. It's hard to have one without the other. Before Felicia, our Diva Advisor, talks about skin care, I want to stress that you can take care of your skin and do it on any budget. When we hear about the $500 jar of face cream that's the latest must-have for our faces, it's tempting to say, "Why bother?" It sounds like skin care is only for the rich. The truth? You can find products that address your skin needs in a range of prices. You'll find them at discount chains like Costco, in-home services like Avon and Mary Kay, drugstores, and exclusive skin salons where there are products that address your skin needs.

Probably the most important thing to take control of is the care of your skin. It's time to bump up your program if you haven't been on one already. Let's start with some professional advice from our in-house esthetician, Felicia.

• Healthy skin requires loving care.

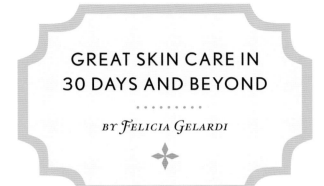

GREAT SKIN CARE IN 30 DAYS AND BEYOND

BY FELICIA GELARDI

Felicia Gelardi is the founder of Felicia Gelardi Skin Care in San Francisco.

1. A month before your dates, schedule two appointments for glycolic peels, two weeks apart. This will exfoliate the skin, removing dead skin cell buildup and leaving your skin brighter. This can keep your skin fresh. It's a good thing to do for yourself every four to six weeks. As an added benefit, skin care products will work better and makeup will go on easier as well.

2. Get your eyebrows waxed and your upper lip waxed too, if you need it. Ask your esthetician to check you out for chin hairs as well, and have them removed. You might not see them, but she will.

3. Assess the products you're using. To keep from getting pigmentation, use rejuvenating products. Vitamin C serum helps build collagen and keeps the skin firm. Products with retinol help with fine lines and wrinkles. Use these from now on.

4. Manicures and pedicures make a world of difference. They look so much better when a professional does them and they last longer too. Getting rid of calluses on the feet does a lot for feeling pretty in sandals.

5. Use sunscreen even when you think you don't need it. Sun damage is cumulative, and one in five people gets skin cancer. Even when it's cloudy and you're only going outside to grab lunch, and especially when you're driving in your car, wear sunscreen. Light coming in through windows still hits your skin and can damage it. Look for titanium dioxide, zinc oxide, or avobenzone as the active ingredient. These protect you against the ultraviolet type B rays of light from the sun (UVB), as well as ultraviolet rays (UV), which are the real culprits when it comes to wrinkles and premature aging. Make sure your sunscreen has an SPF of at least 30. If you're sensitive to the fragrances of these products, keep trying until you find one you like. It's out there. Estheticians stock them as well. Manufacturers are constantly upgrading sunscreens so they aren't sticky, don't leave a residue, and are easier to wear under makeup. Apply it to your face, neck, hands, forearms if uncovered, and if you're wearing an open necked-shirt, apply it to your chest too. Every single day.

6. Get in the habit of daily skin care. In morning and evening, wash your face with a mild cleanser, use a toner, apply vitamin C serum or another serum containing an antioxidant — whatever's appropriate for your skin — sunscreen in the morning only, and then moisturizer.

7.　Toner is important, and it's something that a lot of people don't use because they don't understand its true purpose. Most people think it's used to remove dirt, oil, and other debris from the skin that might be left after cleansing, such as makeup. Not true. There should not be anything on the skin after cleansing (if there is, you're using the wrong cleanser). A toner returns the skin to its proper pH balance after cleansing. It takes the skin about twenty minutes to do that on its own. So unless you want to cleanse, wait twenty minutes, and then apply other stuff, it's wise to use a toner.

8.　Skin can be improved but only if a woman makes a commitment to take care of her skin. There isn't a quick fix. Look at it as a work-in-progress that you and your esthetician approach as a team. It can take a while to figure out what works best for each person. Be patient. It's worth it.

Diva Sense

"My pampering is all about the spa. At a minimum it's a manicure and pedicure, but if I really need a beauty break, I treat myself to a facial and a massage! Also, I use my Sunday nights for a little home spa experience. I exfoliate, do a mask, and apply a deep conditioning treatment to my hair. It's very relaxing, and it forces me to take a little time for myself before I begin another work week."　*Traci*

• Visit your establishment for beautifying skin treatments.

Your Makeup Style

✦ ✦ ✦

Your makeup style should go along with your clothing style. If you have a very relaxed, natural style in your clothes, a natural look in makeup will complement it. If your look is sophisticated, your makeup should look sophisticated too.

Are you Miss Natural? If you're not used to wearing makeup, the smallest amount may make you feel like a streetwalker. You're ultrasensitive to seeing anything on your face. Believe it or not, it's impossible to look natural like you did in your twenties without now using a handful of products. If you haven't been protecting your skin with sunscreen, you could have sun damage. Just evening out your skin tone with a base or foundation that's right for your skin will seem to make you healthier looking instantly. Once you get used to the process of applying your makeup successfully, it will look normal to you. And you'll be getting all these compliments, which will help to reinforce your efforts. If you're just starting, you won't have any bad application habits to get over, a real plus.

If you're makeup shy, you'll at least want to have your eyebrows shaped and choose a lipstick with some sheen. You don't want a matte or brown color. That's too deadening. You want lightness to come to your face. A pale nude eye shadow color all over your eyelids will cover any discoloration. Mascara is a possibility too. You may want some blush. If you know your coloring is cool, look for one in a plum shade. For warm coloring, a peachy color is best. It's all really manageable.

If you're comfortable wearing makeup and you're experienced, then just refining your look may be what's needed for you. I'm going to trust you to have your foundation color checked for shade and texture. You might also want to change your powder blush to a cream one.

Take a look at your lipstick color; you may want to lighten it. Get away from too strong or bold of a lip color. It can be aging. A lipstick with a sheen is more contemporary. If you're using lip liner, be sure we don't see the line separate from your lipstick. A transparent lip pencil can hold your color longer if you have problems with colors bleeding into lines around your mouth. A dab of lip gloss in the middle of your bottom lip will make you feel instantly sexy. It will require reapplying, which is why I don't suggest it for Miss Natural. But you might have the patience for it.

A darkened lid can be aging on a mature woman. Lighten and brighten the lid with light pink, peach, or gold eye shadows. However, frosted eye shadows probably aren't for you. They are easier for young people to wear. Colors with sheen, however, are light reflective and flattering so consider them for all your products. There was a time when it was recommended that women over forty avoid products with sheen. The formulations have been so improved that now it's really a nonissue. If you have hooded eyes, so shadows on the lid can't be seen, add color underneath the eye. A stiff angled brush dipped in shadow can be easier to use than a pencil. Apply the color as close to the base of your eye lashes as possible so it looks natural.

Maybe you wore false eyelashes in high school. That might be over the top now, but false lash separates applied at the outer corner of each eye will give your lashes an upturned look. You don't have to be intimidated; they're easy to use. Go to a makeup counter for guidance.

Stay away from tinted eyeglasses. They cast an unflattering shadow to the eye. You want to eliminate barriers to the eye area other than when you are outside in full sun, and that's when you can whip out your glamorous sunglasses. Your glasses, if you wear them regularly, are your most important accessory, so be sure you keep them updated as well. A dated frame style or one in shiny gold or silver (as opposed to antique or burnished metal frames) will make you look older.

ration dates, and over long periods of time they can become contaminated. You're doing your health a favor by using your products up quickly. The shelf life for mascara is three to six months; moisturizer, three to twelve months; concealers, blushers, and eye shadows are generally good for twelve to eighteen months. If you use products from the health food store, they may have less preservatives in them.

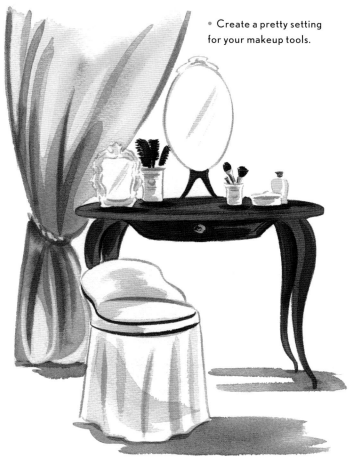

• Create a pretty setting for your makeup tools.

Tool Time

✦ ✦ ✦

Buy and use a magnifying mirror to apply your makeup. Find one with built-in lighting if the lighting is poor where you apply your makeup. That fuzzy eyesight many of us live with can make the application of makeup imprecise. It's so much easier to get that eyebrow line filled in correctly when you can see it!

Having the right brushes is essential to doing a good job at applying products. New ones are always coming out, so find out about what's out there. If you have a girlfriend who is into makeup, ask for some girlfriend time and see what she's got in her makeup kit. We're never too old to have sleepovers, or at least girl time!

I'm giving you permission to dump all those products you've been hanging onto for years. You really only need what you're currently using. Makeup has expi-

See if you can find a "use by" date on the product and dump it when it's time!

When you have fewer things, the whole ritual of putting on your makeup is streamlined. Clear the clutter and then line up your makeup on a tray—how about a silver or crystal one? Lay out the proper products along with the right tools in the order in which you'll be using them. It's amazing how much time this can save each day. You're not fumbling around looking for that one shadow you know is in that drawer somewhere.

Party Makeup

✦ ✦ ✦

When we were young and hanging out on dance floors in clubs until 2:00 a.m, nighttime makeup was more dramatic and made more sense because it helped us to be seen under the strobe lights! Strobe lights are probably not an important consideration now. Your evenings out may be more intimate. You don't need to make dramatic changes to your regimen. You might touch up the makeup you put on earlier in the day, adding more mascara, but don't feel like you're obliged to pull out the sparkly powders and slather them over your collar bones. All of that is a distraction on an older woman. If you're part of the dating scene or you're reinventing yourself as a newly divorced woman, you don't want to look like you're trying too hard.

Another thing that can really take years off our look and give us a confident smile is whiter teeth. As we get older, our teeth can seem to get browner. If we drink red wine, coffee, tea, or sodas, they can dull our chances for a bright smile as well. You might try an over-the-counter teeth whitening product or ask your dental hygienist for suggestions. Bleaching your teeth can make you look younger and healthier. Just don't go crazy with it and get them so white that people around you need to wear sunglasses. That looks too artificial.

Finding Help

✦ ✦ ✦

To find a makeup artist to consult with, ask friends for referrals. When you're meeting friends for lunch and someone is looking fantastic, pull her aside and ask her if she's doing something new, as she looks so great. She may say, "You know, I tried this new product, I've only been using it for a month. Everyone's telling me how good I look. That must be it!" Women will share. (Be sure to check out Resource Day on page 209 in the "Diva Forever" chapter. It's a great way to get your friends to spill the beans about their favorite products and services.)

Another place to get a referral is at better hair salons. They may even have makeup artists in-house. They'll charge a consultation fee, which is well worth it. They'll review the products you're currently using if you ask them, and they'll usually give you a lesson. They may do one side of your face and let you do the other, so you can walk away feeling that yes, you can do it! A makeup demonstration or application at a department store counter isn't a tutorial. A tutorial can give you a lot of confidence. And remember, a makeup artist is an artist. Someone else may do your face differently next week. That's okay. If you like what you see in the mirror, and you've gotten hands-on instruction on how to do this successfully at home, buy the products and start practicing. Your initial investment may seem to be on the steep side, but you'll probably be using these products for a year. Amortized over a year, and then multiplied by all the compliments you're going to get? It's a bargain!

People who offer bridal services will know whom to call for makeup. If you know a wedding planner, ask her to recommend a makeup artist.

Plastic surgeons may have good referrals for medically trained estheticians, dermatologists, and makeup artists.

You can certainly learn things about product and sometimes about technique at cosmetic counters. You might try looking for a salesperson who's close to your age, especially if you like the way her makeup looks on her. Remember, though, she is representing a line, which she hopes to sell to you. You can tell her you want to check out the look of the products on your face at home in your own light before you commit to purchasing anything. Try not to feel pressured. On the other hand, sometimes you find someone who will give you a tip on who produces the best mascara if it's not in their line, and where you might find a better blush.

It's very empowering to learn how to apply makeup that flatters you. It's like anything. It takes good instruction, and with practice, you'll soon feel comfortable and confident.

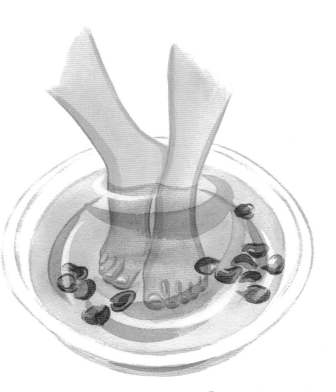

• Treat your feet as well as your face with regular beauty soaks.

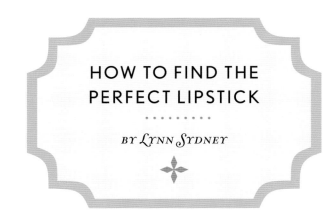

HOW TO FIND THE PERFECT LIPSTICK

BY Lynn Sydney

Lynn Sydney is a makeup artist and style consultant. A former fashion editor, she has written extensively on cosmetics and image.

Finding the right lipstick is an art and a science, but it isn't rocket science. This is the time to ask for help. An experienced consultant at the cosmetics counter of a better department store helps customers select lipstick colors all day. They have loads of practice and can help you too. Here are some useful tips.

1. The very best possible lipstick look always requires more than one product. Mixing two lipstick colors on the lip or using a lip liner underneath a lipstick gives dimension to the color and helps control intensity. (Use the liner to outline and fill in the entire lip.) If a color appears too bright on its own, try using a base lipstick or a lip liner in a slightly darker tone or in a browner tone underneath it to give the total look depth and cut brightness. If a lipstick color is nearly right but feels a bit dark, try adding a dash of nude-beige lipstick on top to tone the lip down. If a color seems a touch dull, try mixing it with a brighter color. If it is really too dull, leave it at the store.

2. Lip color can make teeth look whiter or yellower. Very orange lipsticks in colors like strong apricot and orange-rust will bring out the yellow in teeth. Very purple lipstick colors (violet-pink and purple-burgundy) will also make teeth look yellower because of the high contrast. For the whitest smile, try a neutral pink, peach, or red that's not overly warm or cool.

3. As we mature, shimmery lipsticks look best dotted over a creamy matte lipstick. Worn on their own, a very shimmery shade may settle in lip creases and draw attention to them. Women with silver hair often look great with a touch of shimmer as a top lipstick layer, just don't go it alone.

4. If your favorite lipstick color has been discontinued by the manufacturer, there is a reason. It has dated and it's time to find something better.

5. On some women, lipsticks change color after they are applied. This can be due to the pH of the skin. If colors turn more orangey on you, select a color that looks slightly cooler (a touch more violet) in the tube than what you want. It will warm up on your skin to give you the desired shade. If instead, colors take on a violet cast, select a slightly warmer shade than you want and it will cool down a few moments after application.

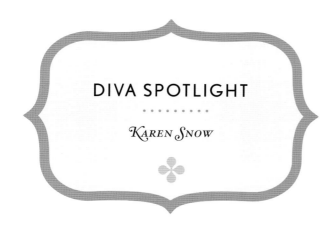

DIVA SPOTLIGHT

KAREN SNOW

I am a forty-nine-year-old romantic at heart with a Scandinavian sensibility and reserve. I have a playful side, and an irreverent wit. I love picnics and tea and music and poetry. I also love to roll up my sleeves and get my hands dirty refinishing furniture, pulling weeds in the garden, oiling a squeaky hinge. I love any project with a noticeable "before and after." Professionally I have been educating men and women in the areas of personal color and style since 1986.

What colors do you wear to flatter your natural coloring?

I love chocolate brown to match my large, doelike eyes. I love tones of pink sand to complement my skin tone. I use touches of soft wood rose to bring out my feminine side.

How do you flatter your assets?

I'm dramatically thin for my height, so I don't mind exposing my bare arms. I love waist details to highlight my small waist.

Name a key diva piece.

A big rectangular Indian cashmere shawl that is almost completely covered with hand embroidery. The color tones are as if you were looking at the Grand Canyon just after sunset. I throw it around my shoulders and I feel yummy.

What are your must-have accessories?

My wedding ring! I still adore it after twenty-one years. Also my very practical and refined gold watch with a small chocolate croc band, heirloom jewelry from my mom and grandmas, and belts when they're in style.

An old favorite that you still wear?

A very old Anne Klein wool sweater, maybe from the late '80s. It has a soft, large cowl neck, is shaped at the waist, and it's in a perfect pale apricot shade that makes my skin look luminous. I get compliments every time I wear it.

Name something you splurged on and never looked back.

A metallic, antique gold leather jacket with ruching at the waist and collar. I throw it on with jeans and a T-shirt and tortoise high-heeled sandals, as well as sand-colored silk crepe pants and jewels.

What's in your underwear drawer?

Three bras (1 beige, 1 cream, 1 black with convertible straps); 12 pairs of brief-style panties; 1 thong (I can't remember the last time I wore it); and 4 sets of long johns, which I use for layering because I'm usually cold. They come in really handy, even under evening wear.

Fashion rules you live by?

I have shoes, bags, and belts in my hair color. They go with everything. I only buy a boot or a sandal, plus a flat and a pump for the season. Then I wear them to death because next year they'll be out of style.

Rules you break?

There's the rule that says "Don't keep anything you haven't worn in two years." I'll keep clothes longer than that. If I absolutely love it and it's classic, it stays in the closet. Part of the game is to see if I can make it fresh and stylish every year. I keep accessories forever, but those that aren't in style I move out of the closet.

Do you have advice you'd like to pass on?

Show up. You are totally unique to the planet. What a gift!

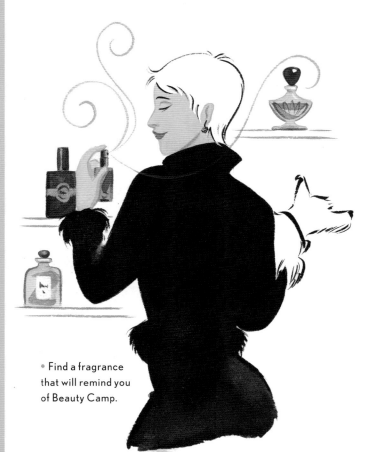

● Find a fragrance that will remind you of Beauty Camp.

How about a beauty soak? Here's something you can do while you're visiting the cosmetics counters this week:

BEAUTY SOAK Scientists say our sense of smell has an indelible memory. We can be in a crowd of people or on a walk in a nature conservatory and a scent will suddenly make us remember a specific moment in our childhood. Instantly, our minds spill out the rich details of that time, just because we caught a whiff of something. I have a friend who chooses a new fragrance when she takes a big trip overseas. She wants to wear that fragrance weeks after the trip and relive her adventures through the scent. Another friend bought a fragrance to wear on her wedding day and during her honeymoon. Later she could relive the love and joy of the commitment she made to her husband throughout their years of marriage. Take some time in the fragrance department of a store and learn about what fragrances you love now. Take home samples. Fall in love with a scent and wear it during your dates. If not perfume, maybe a scented lotion. Months from now when you're wearing that scent, you'll remember these weeks of Beauty Camp when you put yourself first and had fun reinventing your look.

DIVA SENSE

"Don't wear too many scents at one time. Buy unscented beauty products and then you add your own scent. I now layer my scents. I layer three different scents on my chest. If I'm going out to dinner, I don't wear perfume. Too many odors at a dinner table makes you gag." *Debra*

Chapter 14

DIVA DATES

❋

This is the culmination of a project that 30 days ago seemed like a stretch for you. But look! You're here!

You've been through your closet and have it cut back to just your CSF, so you don't have the option of looking bad. All the stuff that didn't fit, wasn't your color, or didn't express you is gone! Poof! You took care of that! Instead, you have beauty bundles that you can grab at a moment's notice if need be. You have more choices with fewer things. And you're wearing what you love! Just think, you used to admire the vintage necklaces you had in your jewelry box. Now you realize you can actually wear them every day! You've updated your hair and makeup, too, and everyone is telling you how great you look.

All that's left for you to do is go out and make your entrance in your three outfits. What a milestone. It's important to celebrate your efforts. Go on those dates, and experience how it feels to be presenting yourself in this new way.

If you find yourself rethinking your outfits at this point, that's okay. Some people make a plan weeks in advance and stick to it. Others make adjustments days, hours, or even minutes before they walk out the door. I invited a few diva pals over to talk about how they put their outfits together. One of them may offer the inspiration you need to make your final decision. Before you make your grand entrance, check out the tips by Diva Advisor Alison Houtte on page 201.

How a Diva Plans an Outfit

✦ ✦ ✦

Mona: "There is usually a feeling or mood that I'd like to convey, and my outfit evolves from there. I usually give it some thought a couple of days in advance to make sure that my accessories are lined up. Once I've decided upon a look, I try it on ahead of time to make sure it's complete. If the outfit is right, I'll have a great time, even if the party is not up to snuff!"

Dija: "Strange as it might seem, sometimes the makeup that I want to wear (either dramatic or natural, for example) is where I'll start. Then I'll take it from there. Sometimes it's my most recent purchase. I just bought a pair of burnt-orange suede sandals, and that was my starting piece. The look was so unexpected

because I kept everything else black and white. I got quite a few remarks!"

Amy: "I go through the rainbow in my head, and see what color strikes me. Sometimes I'm like, 'Wow, I will look *great* in coral tonight' and other times it may be green, black, or whatever. Usually it's a top in that color, and I build from there. I ponder my outfits during my morning spin classes at the gym. It's a way for me to not think about the torture of the class and be happy thinking about clothes."

Cheri: "Since I love shoes and like the way a great pair makes me feel, I will sometimes base an entire date outfit on a pair of shoes I want to wear that day or evening."

Marj: "I almost always zero in on one item I feel like wearing. It might be something I haven't worn in a while and I want to wear it in a different way. It might be a pair of shoes or a piece of jewelry that is fun and fits the mood I'm in. It might also be a brand new item that I've just purchased. I'll wear it three or four times in the same week, experimenting with how it will work with other items in my wardrobe. I guess the big challenge is to have everything in your closet be in textures, fabrics, styles, and colors that you absolutely love. Then it's just the creative side that takes over, like an artist deciding what to include in the picture!"

Karen: "I'll look in the closet and I'll see what tugs at me today. Because I have so few clothes, it's easy for me to run my eyes over everything. Only my things from the current season of the year are visible, including jewelry and shoes. I'll pull one piece that I think I'll feel really good in and then I think, do I need to dress it up or down?"

Focus on the Face

✦ ✦ ✦

As you're reviewing your plans for your date outfits, I want to be sure you've covered a really important point: How are you bringing attention to your face? I want everyone to enjoy your complete outfit, but their eyes should land on your face—the frosting on the cake. Check the list below and be sure at least three items on the list are true of each of your outfits (including makeup and hair). I want to see you, my diva!

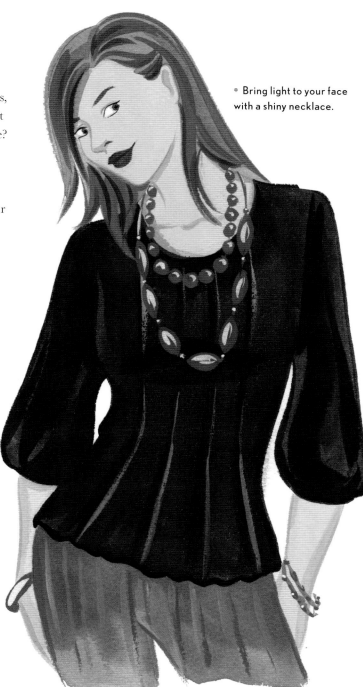

● Bring light to your face with a shiny necklace.

✦ Blush or bronzer is giving definition to your cheekbones, sculpting your face.

✦ Lipstick color is defining your lips.

✦ Your eyebrows are in a defined shape.

✦ The shape of your haircut is bringing attention to your eyes.

✦ Highlights in your hair are bringing attention to your eyes.

✦ Earrings show up and bring light to the face.

✦ An open collar with a necklace nestled inside (more than a simple chain) is bringing color and light to the face.

✦ A contrasting color in the form of an undershirt or a scarf at the neck is bringing attention to the face.

✦ Diamonds at ears or neck (or other material with luster) is capturing light and splashing it up to your face.

✦ Your eyeglasses or sunglasses are bringing the point of attention to your eyes, not your lower cheeks.

✦ A well-fitting turtleneck is bringing attention to your face.

✦ There is detail at the neck of your top or T-shirt—a strip of beads, sequins—that looks like jewels.

✦ The color of your hair is repeated in a piece of clothing, a belt, accessory, shoes, or a coat.

✦ Your eye color is repeated in a piece of clothing, shoes, a belt, handbag, jewelry, a scarf, shawl, or cape.

✦ The collar on a jean jacket (or something similar) is flipped so that it hugs your neck and opens the area near your jaw line, bringing focus to your face.

✦ You are wearing a shawl collar or a collar with body in an unusual shape, opening up the area around your face.

Date Plan and Report

✦ ✦ ✦

Following is space for you to fill in the details of your outfits. Include any reminders like fastening a scarf to a neckline or wearing a brooch in a certain spot under "finishing details." Knowing you've fully worked out each outfit ahead of time will give you the confidence to relax. Add a photo of yourself in each one. When the date is over, report on what worked well, and any adjustments you'd like to make.

Before you go on those dates, however, you'll want to have a dress rehearsal to make sure your outfits are complete (more on that soon). That's a good time to fill in the key style words that your outfit is expressing. Later, when you fill in the report, think about whether the outfit really expressed those words. Sometimes you'll get a comment that will be exactly your style words. "You look so radiant!" Or, "You're so sophisticated and elegant." That's when you know you've really nailed it.

•• Date One ••

Top: ....

Bottom: ....

Jacket: ....

Outerwear: ....

Shoes: ....

Hosiery: ....

Accessories: ....

Handbag: ....

Finishing details: ....

Key style words: ....

Where I'll wear this: ....

REPORT:

How did you feel?

....

....

What worked?

....

....

What didn't?

....

....

What would you do differently?

....

....

....

•• Date Two ••

Top: ....

Bottom: ....

Jacket: ....

Outerwear: ....

Shoes: ....

Hosiery: ....

Accessories: ....

Handbag: ....

Finishing details: ....

Key style words: ....

Where I'll wear this: ....

REPORT:

How did you feel?

....

....

What worked?

....

....

What didn't?

....

....

What would you do differently?

....

....

....

Date Three

Top:

Bottom:

Jacket:

Outerwear:

Shoes:

Hosiery:

Accessories:

Handbag:

Finishing details:

Key style words:

Where I'll wear this:

REPORT:

How did you feel?

What worked?

What didn't?

What would you do differently?

Dressing Up, Dressing Down

✦ ✦ ✦

As one of the divas suggested, it's important to try on each outfit before the date and really go through the full dress rehearsal—foundations and everything. Look yourself over in a full-length mirror. If your outfit needs some dressing up or down depending on where you're going, here are some ways to do that.

To dress up your outfit, try adding one of the following:

1. Sparkly top, scarf, shawl, or handbag

2. Metallic high heels or dressy pumps

3. Dressy jewelry

4. Instead of your regular jeans, wear a pair that's very dark indigo (darker is dressier)

5. Shiny fabric like silk charmeuse

6. Open-toed shoes showing off a fresh pedicure

If you want to dress your outfit down, try adding one of the following:

1. A jean jacket

2. A woven belt

3. Suede boots

4. Woven shoes, like espadrilles

5. A motorcycle type of jacket

6. Non-sparkly shawl or scarf

7. Cotton or linen instead of silk

8. A closed-toe shoe

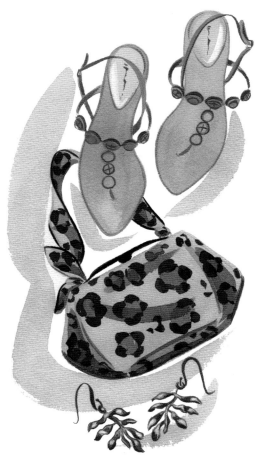

• Dress down an outfit with a fabric bag, sandals (not heels), or a metal earing (no diamond!).

• Dress up an outfit with sparkly clothes or accessories.

Get a Handle on Handbags

✦ ✦ ✦

You won't get out the door without a lecture from me on handbags. There is nothing more frightening than being at a romantic dinner with my sweetheart in an intimate, expensive restaurant when a woman walks in, heading in my direction, with a bag over her shoulder that looks big enough to be a carry-on piece of luggage. I have to duck in order to avoid being walloped by her bag. You think I'm making this up? No, true story.

An evening bag can be smaller than your daytime ones. It doesn't need to carry your full wallet, check-book, and half your makeup. What do you need for maybe 3 hours? Reading glasses so you can read the menu or program. (You might find slim ones in a kiosk at your local mall.) You need your lipstick— not your lipstick gang, just the shade you're wearing. You need a house key or car key, perhaps, but not the full ring of keys. So find a slim key ring for evening purposes. A handkerchief is nice. Bring some cash for a doorman, to tip a valet, or pay for a taxi. Bring one credit card. If you're wearing fancy hosiery, take an extra pair, just in case, wrap it carefully in the handkerchief, and tuck it into your handbag.

Don't make this hard! It really isn't. If you need to, make a list of the bare essentials you need in your purse, and put it in your binder. Refer to it before you go out so you don't have to think. I love work-ing off lists! Better yet, have a handbag beauty bundle started that's just for going out. Make this simple

so you'll do it. Otherwise you're making apologies to everyone about having your big ol' work bag with you. It sends a bad message. Go out! Have fun! You're going on a special date and you're taking a special bag.

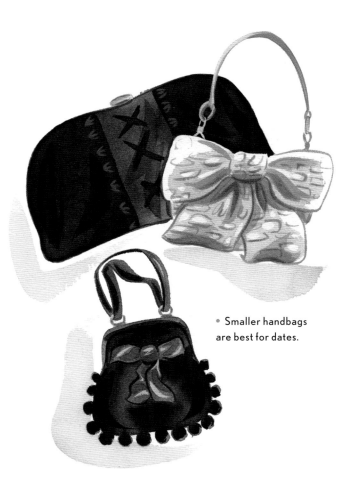

• Smaller handbags are best for dates.

Practice

✦ ✦ ✦

Between now and your actual dates, practice, practice, practice. Practice your new makeup technique every day. You've learned some new things that will feel more natural with practice. Do the same for the products your hairdresser recommended. If necessary, go back to your professionals and ask for a quick refresher course before you go on your dates. One client who'd almost never worn makeup in all of her fifty years learned to apply makeup like a pro. She practiced and asked for extra lessons from a makeup artist until she got it down. She not only looked great, but also felt proud of herself for learning a new skill. She's a college professor and understands the concept of homework. I know that you do too. So if you've learned new skills this month, do your homework and get an A the night of the test—your date night.

Practice wearing your outfit, walking in your shoes, posing for pictures. It's good to find out early that the dress you planned to wear wrinkles horribly the first time you sit down. You still have time to make changes.

Getting Ready

✦ ✦ ✦

The ritual of getting ready to go out and have fun with a sweetheart, family members, or friends is one to be cherished. Aren't we blessed to have these great people in our lives? Slowing down and taking time to enjoy the process of getting ready is a luxury. The way you start the evening, before you've even stepped out of the shower, can enhance your pleasure when you're on your date. Our diva pals have something to say about this. See if they can convince you to take a little extra time and enjoy the process of turning into a diva! Here are their getting-ready rituals:

Traci: "It's all about the music! I literally have a playlist in my iPod that is called 'Getting Ready.' It's full of upbeat music that always makes me happy and is perfect for getting me in the mood to go out on the town."

Kim: "I love starting off with a shower. If I don't have time to take a shower before getting ready, I always feel like something's not right. A clean body to put clothes on, a new palette to start applying makeup—what could be more fun? I love the whole process!! If possible, I allow myself enough time to do things slowly and mindfully. I love watching myself transform right before my eyes."

Sarah: "I love a glass of wine while I am applying my makeup to help me relax for the date."

Colleen: "When I'm getting ready, I have this little silk chemise robe I put on that I feel really special in. I'll get out of the shower, slip into this robe, and wear it while I'm putting on my makeup and doing my hair. I feel elegant in it. It really keeps me in a great mindset."

Tacy: "I'll plan the outfit that morning or the day before. I'll have my nails and pedicure done early in the day; then I'll do a facial and brows. When it's time to get ready, it's country music, candles, hot tea, and lots of lotion all over. I always make sure my feet and legs are soft and pretty no matter where I'm going."

Marj: "The one ritual I have is to always look at myself in a full-length mirror before leaving home or greeting guests. That includes wearing the wrap and handbag. It gives me the total picture of how I will look to others. I've noticed labels hanging out and cat hair on my skirt and fixed them before anyone else noticed them."

• Enjoy the transformation!

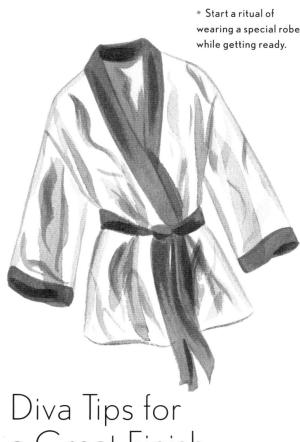

• Start a ritual of wearing a special robe while getting ready.

Diva Tips for a Great Finish

✦ ✦ ✦

I'm trying to think of every last detail so you don't have to. Here are a few last bits of advice I have for finishing your outfits:

1.   Don't look uptight. If you have a tendency to look stiff and uncomfortable, soften up. Have something on that moves—dangly earrings, a bracelet with movable parts or multiple bracelets that slide around on the arm, a skirt with a flippy hemline. Wear a soft handbag. A filmy scarf or cashmere shawl is inviting.

2.   Wear your personal fragrance—but not if you're going to dinner. You don't want your smells to interfere with those of the meal.

3.   Get dressed and then add one thing that looks unexpected. Or make it your secret. I've heard of women who go out with no underwear on because it makes them feel more spontaneous. How about underwear in an outrageously fun color that doesn't show through, but you know it's there? Or put a condom in your handbag, even if you're married. Do something you've never done before.

4.   Express some openness. Wear something that bares a part of you. It could just be an illusion, like a top that is sheer but printed so you see skin underneath, even if it's barely visible. Show off an ankle, wear an open-toe shoe when weather permits, lift your hair off your neck and show your beautiful nape and ears.

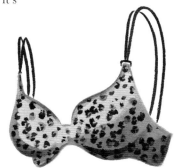

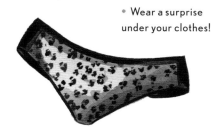

• Wear a surprise under your clothes!

5.   Keep adding to your skills. If makeup is all new to you, start where you can. Lipstick is good. Lipstick and shaped eyebrows are better. Lipstick, shaped eyebrows, and mascara are better yet. The more you blend the products on your face, the more finished and lovely you'll look. You don't have to be perfect, just make a little more effort than you have before.

6.   If you're planning to drape a scarf just so around your shoulders, anchor the scarf to each shoulder with a small safety pin so you can forget about it. Practice this at home first so you know you can be confident and forget about where your scarf is during the evening.

7.   Always take a look at your backside. If you're wearing light-colored clothing, get a second opinion about whether or not your underwear is showing through the fabric. I've seen many patterns of underwear through clothing. Don't let this be you.

8.   Get a great hug from someone before you go out. It will calm you down.

9.   Don't drive in your heels. You don't want to get them scuffed up.

10.   Don't save things for later. Make "later" right now. Pull out the best stuff for your dates. Don't hold back! Life is for living, diva.

11.   Remember, if you're going on a casual date, it doesn't matter if you're the only one who shows up at a football game in heels. If you are really true to yourself and sneakers make you feel like an imposter, don't wear them! Maintain your style. You may look dressed up while everyone else is in jeans and sweatshirts. It doesn't matter.

Wow, there's nothing left to do but say, "Have a blast! You deserve it." You've done your homework. You're ready. Oh, one last thing: Put on the best accessory you have—your smile! When you've completed your dates, come back and join me for some more celebration and fun ideas before we say goodbye.

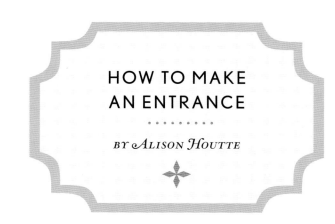

HOW TO MAKE AN ENTRANCE

. . . .

BY *Alison Houtte*

✦

As a former model, Alison Houtte has made many entrances on runways in Europe and New York, and at all those fashionista parties in the Big Apple.

Want to put your best foot forward when you enter a room? Start here.

1. Smile! Even if you aren't feeling particularly great at the moment, show those pearly whites.

2. Feel good about your outfit: Even if you didn't plan your wardrobe until the last minute, and you aren't thrilled with the final result, pretend that you are.

3. Be aware of your posture: shoulders back, chin up (but not so high up that you'll be mistaken for a snob). And please don't ever wear heels you can't walk in confidently. Everyone will notice you, but not for your grace.

4. Wear a great coat: If the weather and event permit, wrap yourself in a layer of velvet, fur, or something else luxurious. Then you can unwrap yourself when you arrive.

5. Don't be too early or too late: Either way, your hostess and the guests will remember you for the wrong reason.

6. Pay attention to the details: If your hair or makeup looks hurried or unfinished, or your shoes need polish or new heels, it will show.

7. Pace yourself: If you feel harried, take a moment to gather yourself before you step into a crowd. Going at a gallop sends the message that you can't relax and just enjoy the party. And never, ever head straight for the bar. That sends the message "I'm a desperate party girl."

8. If the event permits, arrive carrying a bouquet of flowers (for the host or hostess, of course). How can you look anything but great when your face is framed by a bunch of roses or lilies?

9. Take the first step: If introductions are necessary, and no one is making them for you, do it yourself. That shows confidence.

10. Accept a compliment: A grand entrance will quickly fall flat if you dismiss a glowing review with something akin to "Oh, this old rag?" A sincere thank-you is much more effective.

11. Never, ever wear sunglasses indoors. If your eyes look that awful, you should probably stay home.

BEAUTY SOAK You deserve a bouquet of flowers! How about a home delivery? Go online and order an arrangement that's perfect for you. Have them delivered before your first date to honor this exciting finale to Beauty Camp. Or, if you have a favorite florist in town, go out and pick out the bouquet you want. When the florist asks whether it's for someone special, your answer should be *Yes!* Let them wrap it up beautifully. Or, if your best source for flowers is the grocery store, be extravagant. Instead of picking up one bundle of tulips, buy two or three. Create beauty on a grand scale. You are looking forward to your special dates. Your favorite flowers are cheering you on.

• You're looking gorgeous!

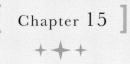

[Chapter 15]

DIVA FOREVER

You're back with tales to tell. How were your dates? How did the grand entrances go? What were the comments? I hope someone took lots of pictures. I suggest you pick out one of your favorites, put it in a pretty frame, and keep it in your dressing area or on your vanity.

The photos make it official. You've graduated from Beauty Camp! Congratulations! Today we'll do some reflecting. I'll also leave you with more ideas for your closet, as I promised, along with several ways you can keep your diva skills sharp.

When you reflect on where you were a month ago, what's different about you now? How about turning to the first tic-tac-toe you made back in chapter 3, which had *ruts* in the center. I bet a few of these (most?) could be crossed off now. They're behind you now. Instead of being a victim of neglect, you've taken charge, made new choices, and gotten a recipe for really looking like yourself. You're a diva! I knew you could do it! Now you can dress to please yourself every day in diva style. I hope you write about your transformation in your journal. I'm sure you have a lot to say.

You've come to the final day—but not the end. The way you learned to honor your color, style, and fit (CSF) can be part of your everyday life. You can pull together an outfit with a star piece and quality support pieces for any occasion. To give yourself more skill and confidence in this area, spend time in front of a mirror when you get dressed. Ask yourself each time what it is you love about your outfit and what's making it work. Describe it. See if you're using your style words. Remember, not every outfit needs to speak to every one of your style words every time. More and more often, though, you'll enjoy getting up in the morning and choosing how you want to feel and look that day. Experiment! Have fun!

What about the days ahead when you really won't have time to play? Well, you'll have a backlog of great outfits that you've already put together. Write them down, just as you did for your dates, and keep those notes in your binder. They'll be your cheat sheets of things that you know work well together. Keep your diva journal in your life. It's a good place to keep track of your ideas, your needs, and your wish list.

You went from dowdy to diva. Just think what else is possible! Do something new to experience yourself in fresh ways. Take a sketch class. Join a garden club. Take Tai Chi. When you experience new things, you keep growing and you don't get stuck in a rut.

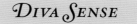

Diva Sense

"I will never be as young as I am today. My face won't look like it does today. It will look different next month, next year, next decade. If there's something about me that I want to put out and celebrate, it better be now. I have a twinge of regret that I didn't celebrate myself earlier. If it means I am overdressed when I go to church on Sundays, oh well. I look like myself. That's more important." *Karen*

Closet Beauty

✦ ✦ ✦

I promised to give you some additional ideas for organizing your closet and storing your clothes and accessories after you cleaned it out. Diva Debra has a great way of storing her necklaces, though they aren't actually in her closet. In her bathroom, a beautiful white Buddha hangs on the wall just to the left of her mirror. Hanging around the Buddha's head are her favorite necklaces. It's so serene.

Create a space for your favorite style icons or for quotes. I cleared a shelf in my closet and keep it decorated with items that remind me of my style. I also have personal mementos there that keep me inspired. I'll rotate them every three months or so. Sometimes I'll gather up small items in the same color when I'm falling in love with a new color.

I've seen women hang large prints of their favorite icons—Jackie O, Coco Chanel, Audrey Hepburn—in their dressing rooms. Big ones! For smaller spaces there are so many wonderful decorative frames that are fashion based. Some have shoes or handbags on them, for example. They're perfect for quotes that remind you to dress as who you are. There have been so many great things said by the divas in this book. Maybe you highlighted some passages. Consider writing them out and having them framed so you can be influenced by them daily.

Create a staging area for you to contemplate or build outfits for upcoming events. One client who loves antiques has an antique brass coat tree in the corner of her bedroom next to her closet. If she's coming

home from work and changing to go out for the evening, she can hang the outfit outside her closet in the morning with the handbag, necklaces, and wraps she intends to wear, along with an alternate. Sometimes we just need more than one choice!

Keep your closet well organized so you can always get dressed in ten minutes. Organize your closet by color and then category of garments (slacks, jackets, tops). It makes it easier to see your clothes. Hang all your clothes on the same type of hanger. If you have the room, keep a professional steamer in there for quick touch-ups.

Make everything as open and visible as possible. Hang jewelry on a belt hanger. Display shoes under the clothes of the same color. Or store shoes on a shoe rack or in clear plastic boxes so they are visible.

• Hang camisoles together on a hanger with multiple hooks.

If you use the shelf above your hanging clothes to store sweaters, T-shirts, jeans, and so forth, put a label below each pile for ease in putting things back. (Use a labeler.) A neat closet will promote creativity. If everything's mixed up and falling all over itself, you'll want to get out of there quickly. Make your closet your shrine to getting dressed.

If you're concerned about repeating outfits at various events attended by the same people, don't depend on your memory. Keep a record of what you wore when in a diary, and keep it in your closet. Or use a hanging calendar. This is especially important if you're in the public eye a lot.

You can also use little Post-its to remind yourself to wear your star pieces. Write the names of star pieces of clothing or accessories that you love on Post-its, one item per Post-it. Scatter them on a calendar. That way, you'll be sure to keep wearing what you love. It's easy to fall into ruts and wear the same thing all the time, neglecting some of your other favorites.

Keep the extra buttons that come with clothing and put them with a sewing kit that you keep in your closet. Get things out of drawers and in hanging closet bags with open shelves when possible. Consider buying a jewelry armoire to keep in or near your closet to store your jewelry. Have bright light in your closet.

I like to use pretty things to store like items. I have round decorative leather containers with lids that hold socks in one, underwear in another. Hatboxes can hold hosiery, shrugs, shawls, and gloves and look pretty, too.

Find ways to customize your dressing area to your liking. An antique desk with a pull-down door could hold your jewelry. For more ideas, go through storage magazines, which you can find on magazine racks in grocery stores or drugstores (they always come out at the beginning of the year). And if you have some empty "nests" in your house, consider turning one into a bona fide dressing room just for you. Go to your favorite boutiques and get ideas about how you'd like to design your space.

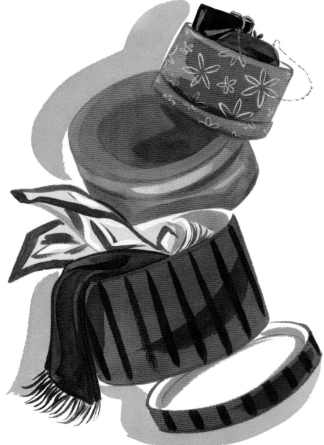

• **Hatboxes are perfect for storing miscellaneous items.**

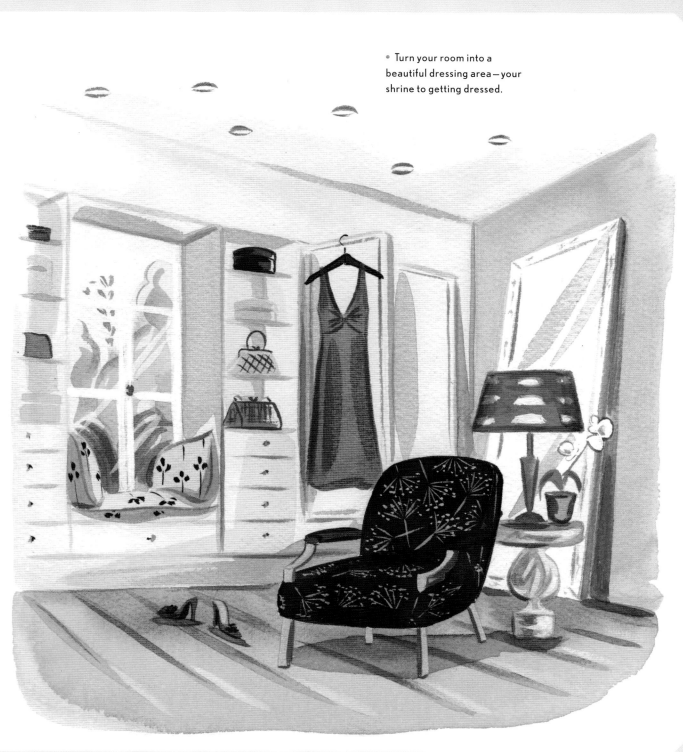

Turn your room into a beautiful dressing area—your shrine to getting dressed.

Manage Your Resources

✦ ✦ ✦

Manage your beauty resources and your beauty notes. Binders can hold a variety of things: your great outfit lists, charts from makeup counters with the makeup design for your face, and your current favorite style photos for inspiration.

Every woman needs a support team. Create a reference page for your wardrobe binder that lists the addresses, hours of service, and phone numbers of the people you depend on for your wardrobe and beauty needs. Keep your resources on one or two pages for easy access. You can do this on the computer on a spreadsheet, or on a simple hand-written list. You can also collect references for services that you haven't gotten around to yet. Consider these services for your list:

1. **Hairstylist.** You want more than one name here in case a special occasion comes up and your primary person isn't able to help you.

2. **Colorist.** This may be someone other than your hairstylist.

3. **Alterations person(s).** Have more than one. Some alterations people will tackle jeans or leather jackets. Others want the simple tasks.

4. **Closet organizer.** He or she can do wonders helping you organize your space if this is challenging for you.

5. **Image consultant.** A personal image consultant can help you meet your style and wardrobe goals, just as a personal trainer helps you meet your physical fitness goals. Word-of-mouth is probably a great way to get names. You can also go to www.aici.org and find a consultant near you.

6. **Dry cleaner.** Know who works quickly and does mending on the spot.

7. **Reweaver.** If moths attack your favorite cashmere sweater, you want this number handy.

8. **Shoe repair.** Keep your shoes and handbags in good repair.

9. **Jewelry repair.** This person will restring your pearls, fix a clasp, or add links to a necklace.

10. **Makeup artist.** She will help you keep up on techniques and products that are especially important to your face now.

11. **Esthetician.** To keep your skin healthy.

12. **Dermatologist.** Get names of good ones for more serious skin care procedures.

13. **Plastic surgeon.** If that's something you're contemplating.

14. **Shopping buddies.** Keep the names of people whom you'd like to invite to shop with you or attend a fashion event with you. Maybe you will become a group like my Bellas. We enjoy talking about fashion, shopping, getting beauty treatments together, and generally encouraging each other to bring out the diva within!

DIVA SENSE

"I was so glad I was ready the day I met my guy on the subway. I was trying to start my life over after my first husband died, and I made sure to do my makeup and get dressed every day. I can honestly say that fashion helped me get through that tough time in my life and saved me in many ways. I don't think a stylish Italian man like my new husband would have tried to get acquainted with a woman with no makeup on, dressed in an ill-fitting sweat suit." *Catherine*

Resource Day

✦ ✦ ✦

I realize you're going to be caught up in your busy life again, but I have a way for you to keep learning about style and beauty while spending time with your friends. It's called Resource Day. The purpose is to share your resources, from beauty tips to the name of your favorite stylist, and much more.

Here's how I organized a Resource Day. I invited friends and friends-of-friends (it's great to have people there that you don't know) to come to my house for a potluck lunch. I asked everyone to bring her °favorite resources in certain categories and gave these important instructions: "Make everything as 'show and tell' as possible. Bring actual stuff and put names and phone numbers of useful people, books, or products on paper. Bring a copy for everybody." Here are some of the categories I used:

1. **Show and tell.** Bring and share your most recent cool "finds."

2. **People bank.** Share the names of people who performed services you were wildly satisfied with. Bring names and phone numbers.

3. **Retail therapy and best buys.** Share places where you've scored great things or particularly enjoy shopping.

4. **Renewal.** Share the names of places where you've been transformed. They can be faraway places, one-day getaways, or things that transform you in an hour, such as musical works, yoga studios, and books.

Five to eight people is plenty. As a result of these exchanges, I've learned where to go to buy beauty products, what new skin care products to try, where to research cosmetic ingredients, and the names of local spas with good discounts. Every day I use some tip or product that I've learned about during a Resource Day. Seriously!

New Fashion Seasons

✦ ✦ ✦

This time next year, you could be wearing something you never thought you'd touch! Perhaps it will be a new color or something that emphasizes a part of your body you've never drawn attention to before. You may find style solutions that you never imagined — that's if you stay open to fashion and what it can give you.

When a new fashion season arrives, your job is to be a style editor. Pick what you like, and leave the rest. Edit the collections, searching for things that seem right for you, and then go try things on. Experiment! Maybe another layer of your personality is ready to bloom! Clothes can help make that happen.

At first, go to stores and shop without your wallet (looking doesn't cost anything). See all the in-store and charity fashion shows you can. The more you view the clothing, the better you can pick them apart and find what you love. Listen to the stirrings of your heart. Is there a color that's calling out to you? Apricot? Lilac? Gold? Teal blue? Is there a part of the body that's being focused on by designers? Maybe sleeves are getting lots of attention. If your arms are among your assets, this could be your special season.

Remember, fashion trends can make us look fresh and youthful when done in the right measure. Youthfulness doesn't mean trying to look like younger folks, but rather, possessing characteristics such as vigor, freshness, or enthusiasm.

You want to be true to your style and avoid becoming a fashion victim, so remember this handy rule of thumb: Take a fashion trend and cut it by about 50 percent. If the young people are wearing platform shoes that are four inches high, make yours two and a half inches high or less. If layers and volume are in, consider half the volume you see on the runway photos. If a model is wearing four trendy things at once, cut it to two and you're doing plenty. It is easy to think of trends as edicts sent down from on high and assume that you have to replace everything in your closet. It's not true. You're in charge.

Trends that you've been through before sometimes return. You'll often hear the line, "If you did it the first time, ignore it the second time." I'm not going to say that. Whenever I do, it comes back to bite me. When I wanted to revolt against the return of leggings, I saw someone my age pulling it off in a way that looked fabulous and totally appropriate. I found a way to wear them again, too. So if you are around to revisit a trend, just approach it differently the second time, maybe with more subtlety. But never say never!

Diva Sense

"I think it's really important to develop a sense of your own aesthetic. It's important to go to art galleries, see beautiful gardens, go to nurseries — to see beauty everywhere. We should be surrounded by beauty. One reason we love clothes is that we love beauty."
Jalyn

Pampering Yourself

✦ ✦ ✦

You set aside time for yourself this month, and you saw a hairdresser and other professionals who made you feel pampered. Hopefully you have a greater appreciation for self care. If you ever feel a little stuck or down in the dumps (it happens to all of us!), or you just need a beauty break, come back to the restorative activities described below. Our diva pals know how to take good care of themselves. Here are the ideas they wanted to share with you:

Helena: "In the past year, I've really made a point to book relaxing appointments for myself. This past week, I went with another girlfriend and had a spa date. We both did an ocean scrub, a massage, and then had lunch. We were able to spend a good part of a day together catching up!"

Elaine: "Every night I relax in a hot bath — no exceptions!"

Anna: "When I need a beauty break from life, I enjoy basking in the sun (using sunscreen, of course) and reading beauty magazines. I also enjoy reading while in a bath of rich oils or salts after a long day. Going to the gym for a long workout with nothing in mind but how good I'm going to feel and look afterward is super-rewarding, as well."

Diana: "For pampering myself I book a facial or a pedicure. If I'm at home with no time for outside services and I need a break, I meditate for twenty minutes or even take a short nap. Both tend to put life back into perspective."

Marj: "The beauty break I've started doing each night is to massage my feet with a wonderful aromatic foot cream before going to bed. The massage relaxes me (an old dancer's trick) and the smell of my lavender foot cream helps me drift off to sleep."

Julie: "My favorite pampering thing is going to my yoga class. It's hard work, but I feel great afterward. Then I come home (it's a night class), pour a glass of wine, and fill up the tub. I light some candles, put on some relaxing music, and have a nice Jacuzzi soak."

Dija: "Pampering comes in the form of my husband's hands. He gives great foot massages and we listen to soothing music. In the summer I love being outside. At night (when there are not too many bugs around), I take a blanket and quite a few candles, light these in the backyard, and have a glass of wine with my husband. It feels like I'm far away and also gives us some alone time and an opportunity to catch up on what's happening in one another's lives."

DIVA SENSE

"Fashion has only one job — to make us beautiful. If it doesn't do that, don't bother." *Christiane*

Divas Never Stop Learning

✦ ✦ ✦

You've heard from a lot of people over these last weeks. You've heard success stories, met some divas, and looked inside their closets. Have you gotten some new ideas? I sure have! Even though I've been in this business for over twenty years, I'm excited about doing some new things.

I'm going to look for more variety in shoes, and make handbags a more fun part of my wardrobe, inspired by Diva Catherine's stash. I want more variety in my life. I'm going to experiment with textured hose and find some glamorous wraps to wear on chilly Sonoma nights. I'm going to keep looking for things in metallic colors; I love the way they make me feel luxurious and I understand that more since hearing from Diva Randi about the healing quality of color. I'm going to pay more attention to vintage jewelry, bags, and coats and bring more unusual pieces into my wardrobe. (Thanks, Diva Melissa!) I'm going to watch more movies from the '50s and take some notes for inspiration. I'm going to create a ritual for skin care, inspired by Diva Felicia's skin care tips. So I guess in some ways, I'm graduating right along with you! It has been a pleasure being with you in Beauty Camp. It has filled my heart every day. Thanks!

Saying Goodbye

✦ ✦ ✦

You know what tickles me? The next time I'm sitting and writing in a coffee shop and an everyday diva walks in, forcing me to stop and stare, she could be you! I'll be admiring how you put those pieces together, how you're wearing your accessories, how you put colors together in such a great way, how you mixed textures and came up with the outfit you did.

What a journey this has been. It's been an honor to be at your side as you've discovered parts of yourself that were hidden from you. I'm sure you've been nervous at times. You probably thought, Can I really look that great? Will it make others uncomfortable if I'm showing up this way? If you spend a day being nervous, and you get out there anyway as your diva self, you'll realize the opposite is actually true. You'll be admired for demonstrating your respect for yourself. Others will want to emulate you. You'll bring smiles to the faces of strangers. You'll inspire others just by being you. That's what divas do. You did it!

Congratulations!
And have fun!

Index

A

Abrie, Colleen, 43-44

Accessories
  benefits of, 109, 110, 142
  classic, 116-17
  editing, 108-9, 110-11
  favorite, 74
  grouping, by color, 112-16
  in outfits, 124
  shopping for, 156-57, 158-59
  vintage, 144-45

Accomplishments, celebrating, 22

AICI (Association of Image Consultants International), 51

Alterations, 161, 208

Ankles, 91

Arms, 86

B

Bags, 156-57, 196

Beauty bundles, 124, 138-43

Beauty Camp
  dress code for, 27
  graduation from, 204
  invitation to, 21
  schedule for, 24, 25-26
  success tips for, 22
  supplies for, 24

Beauty reminder box, 66

Belts, 156

Blue, 59

Blush, 178

Body shape
  acceptance of, 79
  changing, 81
  self-image and, 80-81
  tips for flattering, 83-93

Booty, 89

Boundaries, setting, 22

Bras, 82, 84, 87

Brooches, 116-17

Bustline, 87

C

Calves, 91

Capes, 160

Cellulite, 91

Change, fear of, 13-14

Closet organization, 99-106, 205-6, 208

Clothing. See also Colors; Fit; Outfits; Style
  altering, 161, 208
  duplicates of, 137
  editing, 101-6
  favorite, 74
  outerwear, 160
  ruts in, 40
  sizes of, 81
  star pieces, 123, 129-32, 153-54
  support pieces, 123, 133-37, 161
  underwear, 82, 84, 154
  vintage, 144-45

Coats, 160

Colorists, 208

Colors
  attributes of, 59-60
  benefits of, 49
  contrast and, 52-54
  grouping accessories by, 112-16
  healing properties of, 58
  makeup and, 179
  personal palette of, 50-53, 56-58, 60, 67-72
  ruts in, 50
  style and, 67-72
  warm and cool, 56-57

Concealer, 178

Contrast, 52-54

Cox, Debra, 50, 55

D

Dermatologists, 208

Diva dates

getting ready for, 197-98

handbags for, 196

outfits for, 124-25, 129, 193-94

planning, 26-27, 31-36

practicing for, 197

reporting on, 192-94

tips for, 199-200

Divas

in all shapes and sizes, 11, 21

definition of, 10

examples of, 43-44, 55, 94-95, 120-21, 187-88

Dry cleaners, 208

E

Entrances, making, 201

Estheticians, 208

Exercise, 95

Eyebrows, 178, 180

Eye color, 51

Eyelashes, false, 182-83

Eye shadows, 182

F

Face, focusing on, 191

Facial steam, 76

Fashion seasons, 210

Fear of change, 13-14

Feet, 91

Fit

body parts and, 84-91

for bras and underwear, 82, 84

importance of, 78-79

poor, 82, 103-4

reasons for problems with, 81

Flowers, 202

Fragrances, 188

G

Gelardi, Felicia, 25, 179, 180

Glasses, 156, 183

Gloves, 156

Glycolic peels, 180

Gray hair, 173-74

Green, 59

H

Hair

accepting, 167

caring for, 172

color of, 51

gray, 173-74

ruts in, 168-69

styling, at home, 174

Hairstylists

alternative, 208

booking appointments with, 174-75

finding, 170

working with, 171

Handbags, 156-57, 196

Hips, 90

Hosiery, 156

Houtte, Alison, 201

Houtte, Melissa, 143, 144

I

Image consultants, 208

Immersion, 16-17

Invitations, 37

J

Jewelry

benefits of, 109

classic, 116-17, 118

editing, 110-11

expensive, 118

repairing, 208

ruts in, 40

shopping for, 158-59

size of, 118

Journal, 24

· · **K** · ·

Katayama, Victoria, 74, 75

· · **L** · ·

Lipstick, 182, 186

Litton, Dawn, 167, 171

Lyons, Carole Ann, 12, 13

· · **M** · ·

Makeup

applying, 184

benefits of, 177, 191-92

changes in, 177-78

common mistakes in, 178-79

dumping old, 183-84

help with, 184-85, 208

mirrors and brushes for, 183

nighttime, 184

ruts in, 40, 176

shopping for, 158

style of, 182-83

Manicures, 180

Merzon, Randi, 50, 58

Metallic colors, 59-60

Mirrors, 183

Money, 16

Moving Away From and Moving Toward exercise, 41-42, 99

· · **N** · ·

Neck, 86

· · **O** · ·

Orange, 59

Outerwear, 160

Outfits

accessories in, 124

dressing up or dressing down, 194-95

putting together, 122-28, 138-43, 190

star pieces in, 123, 129-32

support pieces in, 123, 133-37

· · **P** · ·

Pampering, 211

Parties

makeup for, 184

throwing, 37

Patterns, 73

Pear shape, 90

Pedicures, 180

Perfumes, 186

Photographs, 162, 163

Pink, 59

Plastic surgeons, 208

Posture, importance of, 93, 201

Power weapon, secret, 13, 14

Purple, 59

· · **Q** · ·

Quiz, 18-21

· · **R** · ·

Red, 59

Reinventing yourself, 13-14

Resonance book, 46-48, 99

Resource Day, 209

Resources, managing, 208

Reweavers, 208

Roll, 88

Ruching, 88

Ruts, 39-42

in clothing, 40

in colors, 50

in hair, 168-69

in jewelry, 40

in makeup, 40, 176

in shopping, 149

• • S • •

Scalp care, 172

Scarves, 156

Scents, 186

Schuller, Catherine, 81, 83, 94-95

Shapers, 83, 84, 88, 154

Shawls, 156, 160

Shoes, 91, 155-56, 208

Shopping

    for bags, 156-57

    for beauty supplies, 158

    for belts, 156

    buddies for, 208

    experience of, 157-58

    for gloves, 156

    guidelines for, 149-51

    for hosiery, 156

    for jewelry, 158-59

    for outerwear, 160

    for scarves, 156

    scheduling, 152

    for shoes, 155-56

    for star pieces, 153-54

    for sunglasses, 156

    for support pieces, 161

    for underwear, 154

Shoulders, 84

Simmons, Cheryl, 35, 37

Sizes, 81

Skin care, 158, 179-81

Skin tone, 51-52

Sleeves, 86

Sliwa, Cynthia, 116, 117

Snow, Karen, 187-88

Spa day, 75-76

Star pieces, 123, 129-32, 153-54

Style

    color and, 67-72

    defining your, 61-66

Success tips, 22

Sunglasses, 156

Sunscreen, 180

Support, garnering, 22

Support pieces, 123, 133-37, 161

Sydney, Lynn, 186

• • T • •

Teeth, 184

Textures, 73

Thighs, 90

Time management, 16, 24

Toner, 181

Trends, 210

Tummy, 89

• • U • •

Underwear, 82, 84, 154

Untermann, Gloria, 120-21

• • V • •

Vintage items, 144-45

• • W • •

Waist, 88

• • Y • •

Yates, Sunny and Gary, 22

Yellow, 59

Young, staying, 14